Topics in Geriatric Care

Series Editors
Balakrishnan (Kichu) R Nair
School of Medicine and Public Health
Newcastle, Australia

Elizabeth Cobbs
Medicine, George Washington University
Washington, USA

Julie Byles
Hunter Medical Research Institute, University of Newcastle Australia
Callaghan, Australia

This book series draws expertise from across the globe to focus on improving the care of older people in hospital, residential aged care, and general practice settings by adopting an evidence-based approach with person-centered care. The different volumes focus on various aspects of the mind, mobility, medications, multimorbidity of older people to meet their expectations. The role of health services, preventive activities, and treatments in maintaining the quality of life for older people are discussed. Many contributors to the series have contributed significantly to the evolution of curriculum, training, and guidelines in the evolving discipline. All the contributors are leaders in their respective fields.

The series editors are internationally renowned geriatricians and gerontologists. This series will change the approach to the practice of geriatrics.

Elizabeth L. Cobbs • Christina P. Prather
Editors

Diseases of the Mind

Springer

BYWORD BOOKS™

Editors
Elizabeth L. Cobbs
School of Medicine and Health Sciences
Geriatrics and Palliative Medicine
Washington, DC, USA

Christina P. Prather
George Washington Institute for Brain Health and Dementia
Washington, DC, USA

ISSN 2731-5347 ISSN 2731-5355 (electronic)
Topics in Geriatric Care

ISBN 978-981-97-5994-1 ISBN 978-981-97-5995-8 (eBook)
https://doi.org/10.1007/978-981-97-5995-8

This Springer imprint is published by the registered company Springer Nature Singapore Pte Ltd.
The registered company address is: 152 Beach Road, #21-01/04 Gateway East, Singapore 189721, Singapore

Preface

Welcome to a volume about the Mind that touches on more than avoiding dementia, delirium, and depression. Our authors explore a broad spectrum of topics to help practitioners optimize the psychological health and mental well-being of their older adult patients.

To the extent possible, this book is evidence-based, but the evidence base supporting the care of older persons is typically less robust than that for younger persons. The Mind topics reflect many of the geriatric syndromes that influence the brain function of older adults. The chapters are relatively brief but bring up a rich array of dimensions within each section. The opening chapter, "The Normal Aging Brain", provides an evidence-based tour of changes that occur in advancing age. The prevention chapter explores what is known about promoting a healthy ageing brain. The sleep chapter provides a detailed look at the complicated and still mysterious phenomenon of sleep and sleep changes in older persons. From there, you will delve into conditions that often plague older persons, such as mood syndromes, stroke, traumatic brain injury, delirium, and cognitive decline. We also bring you chapters that help understand how older persons can live their best lives in spite of acquiring these conditions.

We hope you will use this book to inform your approach to older persons as the global Age Friendly Movement supports, expands, and promises to help us serve our older patients more effectively than ever before.

Washington, DC, USA Elizabeth L. Cobbs

Introduction to the Series on "Topics in Geriatrics Care"

The population is ageing because of our successful public health measures over the past few decades. Ageing is a global phenomenon. According to the World Health Organization (WHO), 80% of the older people live in middle- to low-income countries. In 2020, the number of people aged 60 years and older outnumbered children younger than 5 years. Moreover, the proportion of the world's population over 60 years will nearly double from 12% to 22%, from 2015 to 2050. Some people describe ageing as a "tsunami", but I differ. Tsunami is unpredictable, but we knew the population was, and is, ageing for several decades. We should have a pro-active, evidence-based approach to ageing and its medical and healthcare needs. With the ageing of the world's population, it has become increasingly important to understand the challenges and opportunities associated with providing high-quality care to older individuals.

WHO has declared the current decade as the decade of Healthy Ageing. So our aim should be to keep the ageing population active, healthy, and happy. In spite of this, ageism is still an issue, both in the wider society and healthcare systems. We know that a majority of older people are independent, in spite of the multimorbidity and chronic diseases. Often an older person is caring for another older person. All healthcare professionals, irrespective of their specialties, should have adequate knowledge in geriatric medicine. Older people suffer from multiple system diseases.

Ageing also is risk factor for frailty. This gives us opportunities to intervene in multiple ways. This series on "Topics in Geriatric Care" is intended to serve as a comprehensive resource for healthcare professionals, researchers, and students around the world who are interested in this field. This series is designed to provide a broad overview of the key topics in geriatric care, with a focus on evidence-based approaches to diagnosis, treatment, and management. It covers a wide range of topics, including the biology of ageing, common geriatric syndromes, psychological issues in ageing, and the social and ethical dimensions of caring for older adults. This series also includes practical information on the assessment and management of common medical conditions in older adults, as well as strategies for promoting healthy ageing and enhancing quality of life. The authors of this series are leading experts in the field of geriatrics, with extensive clinical and research experience with a focus on international best practices and the unique challenges and opportunities associated with providing care to older adults in different parts of the world. Each volume is based on the geriatric syndromes, including what matters to older people, multimorbidity, challenges in the field of dementia, and musculoskeletal health. Often with multimorbidity comes polypharmacy and its consequences. Once an older person gets unwell, they need to get back to their premorbid health with individualized care and rehabilitation.

We hope that this series on geriatrics will serve as a valuable resource for healthcare professionals, researchers, and students around the world, and that it will contribute to the ongoing effort to improve the health and well-being of older adults everywhere.

I am pleased to introduce this volume and the subsequent volumes as the editor-in-chief. I thank the individual volume editors and the staff of Springer Nature for their support.

Balakrishnan (Kichu) R Nair

Contents

The Normal Aging Brain

1

Perry K. Richardson

Key Points

1. Age-related changes are heterogeneous and associated with remodeling through adaptive neuronal plasticity.
2. Healthy adults may develop changes in executive and attentional functions and processing speed, with relative preservation of semantic and verbal knowledge.
3. Systemic factors such as inflammation and gut microbes are likely related to brain function, as are genetic and epigenetic factors.
4. Usual modifiable risk and protective factors do not correlate with the outcome of dementia when tracked in the very old. The presence of senile plaques and neurofibrillary tangles is not predictive of Alzheimer's Disease.

1.1 Introduction

Emerging themes in the medical science of brain aging are that age-related changes associated with functional decline are heterogeneous, not immutable, and are associated with remodeling through adaptive neuronal plasticity.

Not all animals undergo senescence. Among some species, females will reproduce indefinitely, as seen in the Pacific rockfish and sturgeon [1]. Alzheimer's Disease (AD) is not an inevitable outcome of aging, even in advanced age. Despite finding pathological evidence of senile plaques and neurofibrillary tangles in normal-aged brains and those with AD, the presence of these findings is not predictive

P. K. Richardson (✉)
Department of Neurology and Rehabilitation Medicine, George Washington University, Washington, DC, USA
e-mail: prichardson@mfa.gwu.edu

E. L. Cobbs, C. P. Prather (eds.), *Diseases of the Mind*, Topics in Geriatric Care,
https://doi.org/10.1007/978-981-97-5995-8_1

of AD. The risk of AD is actually reduced in those over 90 compared to ages 60–80 [2].

1.2 Neurocognitive Changes in Normal Aging

Healthy adults may develop changes in executive and attentional functions and processing speed, with relative preservation of semantic and verbal knowledge. Semantic memory refers to meaning, understanding, and general knowledge and remains stable with a later-life decline. Episodic and working memory, considered the interface between attention focusing, retrieval, and long-term memory, may decline steadily from early adulthood. Cognitive patterns can be divided into resilient "crystallized intelligence" (skills, abilities, and knowledge) and changeable "fluid intelligence" (problem-solving and reasoning). Since crystallized intelligence is due to accumulated information over time, older adults tend to perform better at tasks requiring crystallized intelligence than younger adults. Fluid cognition includes the innate ability to process and learn new information, solve problems, and attend to and manipulate one's environment, such as orienting and navigating [3]. These changes in healthy aging are contrasted with those of AD, where cognition is characterized by notably impaired memory and semantic and verbal abilities. Cohort studies suggest cognitive changes begin in the 1930s, while longitudinal studies that identify change occurring later (1960s) may mask decline due to retest effects [4].

1.3 Structural Brain Changes in Aging

Gray matter volume declines after age 20, with steadily progressive atrophy in the prefrontal cortex, hippocampus, insula, putamen and caudate, thalamus, superior parietal and inferior temporal areas. Accelerated atrophy occurs over age 70, especially in the hippocampus. Healthy older persons have decelerated atrophy in the prefrontal cortex and relative preservation of the entorhinal cortex. The reduced volume is due to more reduced synaptic density, dendritic length and arborization, and neuronal size than to neuron loss [5, 6].

White matter volume decreases with a U-shaped curve [7], increasing until age 50, then declining, affecting multiple areas. Changes are shown graphically in Fig. 1.1 [8]. There is relatively little known about sex differences in human brain structure with normal aging [9].

In normal aging, gray matter volume change predominates in the frontal lobe, with an anterior–posterior gradient as compared to hippocampal atrophy and posterior–anterior gradient in AD. White and gray matter atrophy is similar in normal aging, but the gray matter is markedly greater in AD.

Senile plaques and neurofibrillary tangles (NFT) are found in healthy aged brains, with distribution more narrowly restricted to the hippocampus, as opposed to more widespread deposition occurring in the entorhinal cortex in AD. In the

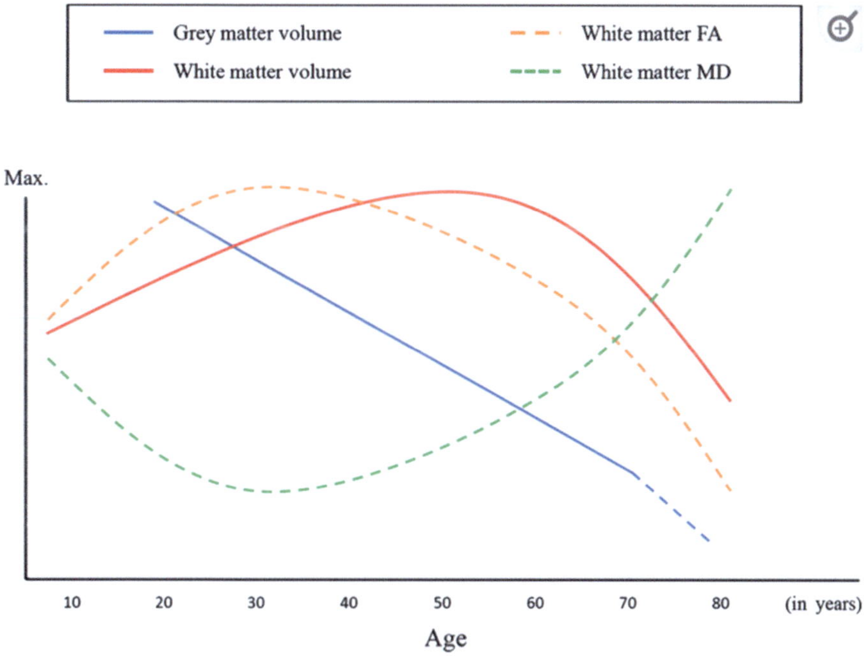

Fig. 1.1 Hypothetical model of global structural cerebral changes across the lifespan (particularly based upon the results of Good et al. and Westlye et al.). The diagram illustrates the different patterns of changes in grey matter volume, white matter volume, and white matter integrity (FA, fractional anisotropy; MD, mean diffusivity). [Reprinted from J Alzheimers Dis, 57(2), Toepper M. Dissociating Normal Aging from Alzheimer's Disease: A View from Cognitive Neuroscience, pp. 331–352, Copyright 2017, with permission from IOS Press. The publication is available at IOS Press through https://doi.org/10.3233/JAD-161099]

oldest AD patients, i.e., those with delayed onset, a relatively lower neuronal loss and burden of NFTs has been reported. Instead, mean capillary diameter reportedly better correlates with cognitive changes in those over 90, suggesting that AD pathology is not a mandatory phenomenon of increasing age [10].

1.4 Functional Brain Changes in Aging

Functional changes are demonstrated using functional MRI (fMRI), electroencephalography, or magnetoencephalography. Prefrontal cortex activation [11] and anterior–posterior connectivity [12] are reduced in healthy older adults, with some reports of bilateral frontal activation or relative suppression of hemispheric activation [13]. Whether these patterns represent impairment, compensation, or even increased functional efficiency (cognitive reserve) is unsettled. Neurotransmitter changes in healthy older adults show reduced dopamine receptor density [14], which is correlated with reduced processing speed and working memory [15].

Cerebral activation studies show a posterior to anterior shift in normal aging, but in AD, they show more parietal than a frontal response to increasing task load. Functional connectivity impairment affects frontostriatal connections in normal aging and hippocampal connections in AD. Finally, neurotransmitter dysfunction affects dopamine circuits in healthy aging and acetylcholine circuits in AD.

Research on astroglial cells, the supporting system for neurons, has demonstrated functional and morphological change with healthy aging and degenerative disease, contributing to the reduced transmitter and ion clearance, dwindling neurogenesis, and repair.

1.5 Adaptive Brain Changes in Normal Aging

While neurogenesis declines with age, those neurons produced are identical dendritically to those formed in the young. Studies show a correlation between reduced hippocampal neurogenesis and memory loss [16]. In mice, an enriched environment was shown to correlate with increased neurogenesis [17], which may imply psychological and social cofactors for brain health. Recently, the Klotho gene, which, among other things, regulates phosphate and calcium metabolism, has been found to protect against oxidative stress and apoptosis, potentially improving white matter integrity through inhibition of insulin-like growth factor-1 (IGF-1) [18].

Of the so-called Pillars of Aging (metabolism, stress adaptation, stem cells and regeneration, proteostasis, macromolecular damage, epigenetics, and inflammation) that can have an effect on cognitive aging, inflammation is increasingly being linked to aging and chronic disease. The basal inflammatory response rises with age, leading to low-level chronic inflammation that is likely maladaptive, promoting aging and disease.

Not all older persons suffer from age-related diseases. Centenarians who appear to defy aging have a large quantity of circulating anti-inflammatory molecules [19]. These oldest old show a complex and heterogeneous phenotype determined by an improved ability to adapt and remodel in response to physical and chemical agents, psychological stress, and biological stimuli such as viral, bacterial, and tumor antigens [20].

Immunosenescence likely reflects a mix of adaptive/resilience and maladaptation [21]. Older people are characterized by extreme heterogeneity due to the numerous and different exposure factors encountered lifelong that can determine each individual's different immune responses (immunobiography) [22].

Microbes in the gut (GM) influence the immune system, and alteration from various factors can promote inflammation. Diet, geography, physical activity, and other factors may swing the pro-inflammatory/anti-inflammatory balance [23]. A study of GM from centenarians found some possibly protective species. It reported a higher prevalence of *Bifidobacterium*, a long time a known probiotic group of bacteria, as well as higher abundances of subdominant members of the human gut ecosystem that have been explored only recently, such as *Akkermansia* and *Christensenellaceae*, which may contribute to immune response [24].

1.6 Genetics of Healthy Aging and Longevity

Molecular genetics has led to the discovery of heritable contributors to intelligence, cognitive function, and disease. Genome-wide association studies identify novel disease genes; however, environmental and epigenetic factors are significant for aging brain health and longevity. Twin studies have shown that general intelligence hereditability increases with age to about 62% by age 7–10 [25], yet the concordance rate for AD among identical twins is only 60% [26].

The best-known disease risk gene is the association of apolipoprotein E gene with the epsilon-4 genotype (ApoE-ε4) with AD. Inheritance of two ε4 alleles increases the risk of developing AD, while heterozygotes and those carrying the ε2 allele show less risk. Studies on apparently non-demented aged subjects with the APOE-ε4 allele have shown qualitative negative changes in visuospatial attention [27]. Other gene polymorphisms associated with aspects of cognition include those related to dopamine availability and metabolism (COMT, dopamine beta-hydroxylase) or acetylcholine (CHNRA4) [28]. Yet, the majority of ε4 carriers do not go on to develop AD. In the longitudinal Nun Study, the activity logs of 801 clergy were correlated with the development of AD ($N = 111$) followed over an average of 4.5 years. Increased activity level, including intellectual engagement, was associated with decreased risk of AD, this was independent of APOE allele status [29]. Other studies indicate physical and cognitive activities reduced later incidence of AD more strongly in APOE ε4 carriers.

Modifiable risk and protective factors do not correlate with the outcome of dementia when tracked in the very old. A subgroup of 278 subjects over 85 years old from the Cambridge over-75s Cohort Study was followed until death. Modifiable risk factors, including diabetes, depression, coronary heart disease, hypertension, alcohol consumption, smoking status, physical activity, and cognitive activity, did not show predictive power for the development of dementia in the very old. This may explain the variability in the results of lifestyle interventions in some studies, suggesting that interventions may be more effective when directed earlier in life [30, 31].

The genetics of longevity is a rapidly advancing area, actualizing a “positive biology” [32] with the potential for therapeutic intervention. The APOE gene, FOXO3A gene, Progeria, telomere maintenance, and DNA methylation genes have been linked to longevity [33]. These discoveries support the theory of a mechanism for “buffering” frailty alleles despite the retention of common disease gene variants [34].

We have always known that the brain is unique. As a post-mitotic organ, it cannot be renewed like skin or gut, yet the persistence of neurons for 80-plus years confers the ability to preserve memories and other learned functions. The gracious aging of the brain was noted in one of the first longitudinal investigations of nearly 900 subjects over age 80, including 74 centenarians, published in Cambridge in 1889. The author, George Murray Humphry, concluded: “Indeed, the brain in many held out as well or better than other organs—which may be regarded one of the bright rays, if not the brightest, in the centenarian landscape” [35].

References

1. Finch C. Longevity, senescence and the genome. University of Chicago Press; 1990.
2. Rebeck GW, et al. Reduced apolipoprotein epsilon 4 allele frequency in the oldest old Alzheimer's patients and cognitively normal individuals. Neurology. 1994;44(8):1513–6.
3. Elias L, Saucier D. Neuropsychology: clinical and experimental foundations. Boston: Pearson Education; 2006.
4. Salthouse TA. When does age-related cognitive decline begin? Neurobiol Aging. 2009;30(4):507–14.
5. Fjell AM, Walhovd KB. Structural brain changes in aging: courses, causes and cognitive consequences. Rev Neurosci. 2010;21(3):187–221.
6. Storsve AB, et al. Differential longitudinal changes in cortical thickness, surface area and volume across the adult life span: regions of accelerating and decelerating change. J Neurosci. 2014;34(25):8488–98.
7. Westlye LT, et al. Life-span changes of the human brain white matter: diffusion tensor imaging (DTI) and volumetry. Cereb Cortex. 2010;20(9):2055–68.
8. Toepper M. Dissociating normal aging from Alzheimer's disease: a view from cognitive neuroscience. J Alzheimers Dis. 2017;57(2):331–52.
9. Ruigrok AN, et al. A meta-analysis of sex differences in human brain structure. Neurosci Biobehav Rev. 2014;39:34–50.
10. Imhof A, et al. Morphological substrates of cognitive decline in nonagenarians and centenarians: a new paradigm? J Neurol Sci. 2007;257(1–2):72–9.
11. Reuter-Lorenz P. New visions of the aging mind and brain. Trends Cogn Sci. 2002;6(9):394.
12. Nagel IE, et al. Load modulation of BOLD response and connectivity predicts working memory performance in younger and older adults. J Cogn Neurosci. 2011;23(8):2030–45.
13. Cabeza R. Hemispheric asymmetry reduction in older adults: the HAROLD model. Psychol Aging. 2002;17(1):85–100.
14. Backman L, et al. The correlative triad among aging, dopamine, and cognition: current status and future prospects. Neurosci Biobehav Rev. 2006;30(6):791–807.
15. Li SC, Lindenberger U, Backman L. Dopaminergic modulation of cognition across the life span. Neurosci Biobehav Rev. 2010;34(5):625–30.
16. Isaev NK, Stelmashook EV, Genrikhs EE. Neurogenesis and brain aging. Rev Neurosci. 2019;30(6):573–80.
17. Kempermann G, Gast D, Gage FH. Neuroplasticity in old age: sustained fivefold induction of hippocampal neurogenesis by long-term environmental enrichment. Ann Neurol. 2002;52(2):135–43.
18. Duce JA, et al. Gene profile analysis implicates Klotho as an important contributor to aging changes in brain white matter of the rhesus monkey. Glia. 2008;56(1):106–17.
19. Sizzano F, et al. Evaluation of lymphocyte response to the induced oxidative stress in a cohort of ageing subjects, including semisupercentenarians and their offspring. Mediat Inflamm. 2018;2018:7109312.
20. Franceschi C, et al. Centenarians as a 21st century healthy aging model: a legacy of humanity and the need for a world-wide consortium (WWC100+). Mech Ageing Dev. 2017;165(Pt B):55–8.
21. Fulop T, et al. Immunosenescence is both functional/adaptive and dysfunctional/maladaptive. Semin Immunopathol. 2020;42(5):521–36.
22. Franceschi C, et al. Immunobiography and the heterogeneity of immune responses in the elderly: a focus on inflammaging and trained immunity. Front Immunol. 2017;8:982.
23. Santoro A, et al. Inflammaging, hormesis and the rationale for anti-aging strategies. Ageing Res Rev. 2020;64:101142.
24. Biagi E, et al. Gut microbiota and extreme longevity. Curr Biol. 2016;26(11):1480–5.

25. Davis OS, Haworth CM, Plomin R. Dramatic increase in heritability of cognitive development from early to middle childhood: an 8-year longitudinal study of 8,700 pairs of twins. Psychol Sci. 2009;20(10):1301–8.
26. Gatz M, et al. Role of genes and environments for explaining Alzheimer disease. Arch Gen Psychiatry. 2006;63(2):168–74.
27. Greenwood PM, et al. Genetics and visual attention: selective deficits in healthy adult carriers of the epsilon 4 allele of the apolipoprotein E gene. Proc Natl Acad Sci U S A. 2000;97(21):11661–6.
28. Green AE, et al. Using genetic data in cognitive neuroscience: from growing pains to genuine insights. Nat Rev Neurosci. 2008;9(9):710–20.
29. Wilson RS, et al. Participation in cognitively stimulating activities and risk of incident Alzheimer disease. JAMA. 2002;287(6):742–8.
30. Deckers K, et al. Lack of associations between modifiable risk factors and dementia in the very old: findings from the Cambridge City over-75s cohort study. Aging Ment Health. 2018;22(10):1272–8.
31. Pekkala T, et al. Development of a late-life dementia prediction index with supervised machine learning in the population-based CAIDE study. J Alzheimers Dis. 2017;55(3):1055–67.
32. Farrelly C. 'Positive biology' as a new paradigm for the medical sciences. Focusing on people who live long, happy, healthy lives might hold the key to improving human well-being. EMBO Rep. 2012;13(3):186–8.
33. Brooks-Wilson AR. Genetics of healthy aging and longevity. Hum Genet. 2013;132(12):1323–38.
34. Bergman A, et al. Buffering mechanisms in aging: a systems approach toward uncovering the genetic component of aging. PLoS Comput Biol. 2007;3(8):e170.
35. Humphry GM. Old age: the results of information received respecting nearly nine hundred persons who had attained the age of eighty years. Cambridge: Macmillan and Bowes; 1889.

Preventive Health and Promoting a Healthy Aging Brain

2

Hannah Fine, Leila El-Badry, and Mikhail Kogan

Key Points

1. Optimizing brain health requires a multimodal approach.
2. A healthy lifestyle encompasses several elements key to brain health.
3. Physical and cognitive exercises are essential to long-term brain health.
4. Optimizing cardiovascular health and physiologic stress can reduce the risk of dementia and late-life cognitive loss.

2.1 Introduction

A comprehensive, multifaceted approach promotes brain health in later life. Across the world, in regions called Blue Zones, record numbers of people live to 100 years of age. Despite advanced age, which is typically a nonmodifiable risk factor for developing Alzheimer's Disease (AD), the incidence of AD in these regions is very low [1]. Individuals from these regions characteristically have healthy lifestyles and overall good health. A healthy lifestyle can decrease the risk of dementia regardless of genetics.

H. Fine
George Washington University, Washington, DC, USA

L. El-Badry
Washington University in St. Louis, St. Louis, MO, USA

M. Kogan (✉)
Center for Integrative Medicine, George Washington University, Washington, DC, USA
e-mail: mkogan@mfa.gwu.edu

E. L. Cobbs, C. P. Prather (eds.), *Diseases of the Mind*, Topics in Geriatric Care,
https://doi.org/10.1007/978-981-97-5995-8_2

2.2 Environmental Risk Factors and Prevention Targets

Many environmental factors increase the risk for cognitive decline, and frequent exposure may increase the risk for cognitive decline or dementia. Chronic exposure to toxic metals and chemicals like aluminum, lead, mercury, extremely low-frequency electromagnetic fields, or organophosphate pesticides may play a role in the development and progression of the disease [2–5]. Mold toxicity is another factor correlated with the development of AD [3].

Chronic physiologic stress due to frequent stress exposure contributes to increased dementia incidence in low-income communities [6]. These communities also experience reduced access to healthful foods and increased health risks due to proximity to densely polluted areas [7]. These factors contribute negatively to many health conditions, including dementia.

Studies show that there is an increased risk for dementia and symptom severity in Black Americans [8]. One explanation may be that Black Americans have a higher allostatic load compared to non-Hispanic white American counterparts [9]. Allostatic load refers to the cumulative burden of chronic stress and life events surpassing one's coping capacity.

2.3 Modifiable Risk Factors for Brain Health

2.3.1 Chronic Inflammation and Physiologic Stress

Stress, via the hypothalamic-pituitary axis (HPA), increases the risk for cognitive decline directly by causing neurotoxic damage to cells in the hippocampus [10]. It is also associated with AD risk factors of inflammation, calcium dysregulation, depression, and sleep deprivation [11]. Stress can affect one's risk for AD indirectly by increasing the risk and exacerbation of other medical conditions. When there is a concern for chronic stress, assessing the cortisol level is clinically relevant to measure HPA function and drive clinical interventions targeted at physiologic stress reduction.

2.3.2 Gut–Brain Axis

Accumulating research on the gut microbiome and gut–brain axis demonstrates that gut dysbiosis can cause or exacerbate cognitive concerns [11]. Insufficient amounts of *Bacteroides* and an overabundance of other microbes in the gut can be significant risk factors for dementia [12].

2.3.3 Sleep

Negative sleep changes may be linked to early-stage cognitive decline and dementia. Obstructive sleep apnea and prolonged or shortened sleep duration are all risk factors for AD [13]. OSA may exacerbate AD risk by causing oxidative stress in periods of hypoxia and worsening cardiovascular comorbidities, along with disruptions in sleep [13]. Inadequate sleep increases dementia risk through reduced ability for deep NREM sleep brain waves to transport memories from the hippocampus to more permanent storage sites. Additionally, the clearance of β-amyloid, which is produced during the day and cleared during sleep, may be reduced when sleep is disrupted [14]. Lastly, impaired circadian rhythm also contributes to sleep quality and cognition. When counselling patients, optimal sleep duration has been shown to be 7–8 h.

2.3.4 Oral Health

Poor oral health may pose a risk for AD. Various factors contribute, including nutritional deficit from improper mastication, amalgams containing mercury, and oral dysbiosis [15]. Overgrowth of the bacteria, *P. gingivalis*, can lead to periodontal disease and chronic low-grade inflammation and can even transmigrate to the brain if untreated [16].

2.3.5 Cardiovascular Health

Vascular risk factors for cognitive decline include hypertension, hyperlipidemia, obesity, and diabetes. Reduction of high blood pressure is thought to be neuroprotective.

2.4 Nutrition and Brain Health

Anti-inflammatory diets have all had some evidence for a protective effect against AD. A Mediterranean diet is rich in B vitamins, folic acid, and omega-3s, which all promote anti-inflammatory and anti-oxidative effects [17]. The MIND diet, which combines the Mediterranean diet and the DASH diet, has also shown protective effects, lowering the risk for AD by 53% [18]. Intermittent fasting (IF) can be helpful in preventing cognitive decline. IF has been shown to reduce inflammation and oxidative damage and has a neuroprotective effect during ketogenesis [19]. The KetoFLEX diet comes from the ReCODE protocol and supports ketogenesis, sources a variety of different food types, reduces meat intake, and promotes IF [20].

Increased fish consumption reduces AD risk according to epidemiological data [21, 22]. This is likely because DHA, EPA, and ALA contribute to cell membrane viscosity and the anti-inflammatory response [23]. While adequate fish intake is advised for promoting a healthy brain, it is important to make sure the fish consumed is not high in mercury, which has become a common issue.

2.4.1 Healthy Brain Diet

- Majority intake: fresh fruits and vegetables, antioxidant rich foods (berries, turmeric, and green tea).
- ↑ Low-glycemic index foods.
- ↑ Dietary omega-3 fatty acids.
- ↓ Proinflammatory foods (red meat, dairy, and sugar).
- Overnight fasting for ketogenesis.

2.5 Physical and Cognitive Exercise

Aerobic exercise improves cognition in healthy individuals [24]. Exercise has anti-oxidative and anti-inflammatory effects and helps to control comorbidities like diabetes or hypertension [25]. Further, exercise has been shown to increase gene expression relating to mitochondrial health and synaptic plasticity, as well as decrease extracellular amyloid plaques in the hippocampus and frontal cortex [25–27]. Exercising for 30–60 min 5×/weekly helps to maintain healthy cognition and prevents cognitive decline [28].

Yoga and tai chi are movement practices that also have spiritual and psychological benefits. These mind-body practices improve stress levels and cognition [29, 30].

Cognitive training helps maintain cognition but remains underutilized. Participating in activities that engage the brain, like playing board games, reading, playing music, or learning a language, is highly recommended for preventing cognitive decline. Existing evidence indicates that musicians generally outperform non-musicians in cognition and have a significantly reduced risk of dementia [31].

2.6 Meditation, Spirituality, and Purpose

Growing research confirms the neuroprotective effects of meditation. One study showed that the brains of long-term meditators on MRI appeared 7.5 years younger than controls at age 50 [32]. Meditation enhances emotional regulation via fronto-limbic networks and can help retain neural structure and function [33]. Practicing mindfulness-based stress reduction (MSBR) increases telomerase, reduces depressive symptoms, and improves subjective sleep quality [34]. Furthermore, MBSR may prevent neuronal loss by increasing the neuronal expression of miR-29c, which inhibits the expression of genes that cause neuronal death [35].

Spirituality is any self-defined, personal connection with a religious and/or transcendental practice, institutional or otherwise [36]. Aspects of spirituality that incorporate healthy practices for the mind-body positively influence mental health and stress levels [36].

Maintaining a healthy brain involves having a well-founded sense of purpose. An overarching personal intention can help to motivate one in their daily life and promote good mental health [37].

2.7 Summary

A comprehensive, multimodal approach to brain health minimizes risk factors and optimizes opportunities for cognitive health. While the implementation of genetic-based multimodal prevention programs like RECODE is likely to remain restricted to memory care centers and limited due to complexity, access, and cost, many of the modalities mentioned can be safely advised upon by providers and implemented by patients committed to long-term healthy brain aging.

Diet	• Anti-inflammatory, Mediterranean, MIND, KetoFLEX
	• High intake: Plant-based, high-antioxidant foods (green leafy vegetables, turmeric, berries, green tea, etc.)
Exercise/training	• Physical 30 min/day
	• Cognitive 30 min/day
Mind-body/stress reduction	• Mind-body practice 15–30 min/day
	• Maintain a sense of life purpose
	– Can manifest in many ways (spirituality, passion, volunteerism, purposeful engagement)
Lifestyle risk factors	• Avoid smoking and excessive alcohol consumption
	• Prevent/control metabolic disorders
Supplementation	• Consider high-quality methylated B-complex for patients 65+
	• Patients on low-fat diets can take fish oil supplements

References

1. Buettner D. The blue zones challenge: a 4-week plan for a longer, better life. National Geographic Society; 2021.
2. Rondeau V, Jacqmin-Gadda H, Commenges D, Helmer C, Dartigues JF. Aluminum and silica in drinking water and the risk of Alzheimer's disease or cognitive decline: findings from 15-year follow-up of the PAQUID cohort. Am J Epidemiol. 2009;169(4):489–96. https://doi.org/10.1093/aje/kwn348.
3. Vasefi M, Ghaboolian-Zare E, Abedelwahab H, Osu A. Environmental toxins and Alzheimer's disease progression. Neurochem Int. 2020;141:104852. https://doi.org/10.1016/j.neuint.2020.104852.
4. Kamel F, Hoppin JA. Association of pesticide Exposure with neurologic dysfunction and disease. Environ Health Perspect. 2004;112(9):950–8. https://doi.org/10.1289/ehp.7135.
5. Jalilian H, Teshnizi SH, Röösli M, Neghab M. Occupational exposure to extremely low frequency magnetic fields and risk of Alzheimer disease: a systematic review and meta-analysis. Neurotoxicology. 2018;69:242–52.

6. Balls-Berry JJE, Babulal GM. Health disparities in dementia. Continuum (Minneapolis, Minn). 2022;28(3):872–84. https://doi.org/10.1212/CON.0000000000001088.
7. Baum A, Garofalo JP, Yali AM. Socioeconomic status and chronic stress: does stress account for SES effects on health? Ann N Y Acad Sci. 1999;896(1):131–44. https://doi.org/10.1111/j.1749-6632.1999.tb08111.x.
8. Lennon JC, Aita SL, Bene VAD, et al. Black and White individuals differ in dementia prevalence, risk factors, and symptomatic presentation. Alzheimers Dement. 2022;18(8):1461–71. https://doi.org/10.1002/alz.12509.
9. Geronimus AT, Hicken M, Keene D, Bound J. "Weathering" and age patterns of allostatic load scores among blacks and whites in the United States. Am J Public Health. 2006;96(5):826–33.
10. Rothman SM, Mattson MP. Adverse stress, hippocampal networks, and Alzheimer's disease. NeuroMolecular Med. 2010;12(1):56–70. https://doi.org/10.1007/s12017-009-8107-9.
11. Khalsa DS. Stress, meditation, and Alzheimer's disease prevention: where the evidence stands. J Alzheimers Dis. 48(1):1–12. https://doi.org/10.3233/JAD-142766.
12. Almeida C, Oliveira R, Soares R, Barata P. Influence of gut microbiota dysbiosis on brain function: a systematic review. Porto Biomed J. 2020;5(2):1–8. https://doi.org/10.1097/j.pbj.0000000000000059.
13. Cooke JR, Ancoli-Israel S, Liu L, et al. Continuous positive airway pressure deepens sleep in patients with Alzheimer's disease and obstructive sleep apnea. Sleep Med. 2009;10(10):1101–6. https://doi.org/10.1016/j.sleep.2008.12.016.
14. Nedergaard M, Goldman SA. Glymphatic failure as a final common pathway to dementia. Science. 2020;370(6512):50–6. https://doi.org/10.1126/science.abb8739.
15. Popovac A, Čelebić A, Peršić S, Stefanova E, Lemić AM, Stančić I. Oral health status and nutritional habits as predictors for developing Alzheimer's disease. Med Princ Pract. 2021;30(5):448–54. https://doi.org/10.1159/000518258.
16. Dominy SS, Lynch C, Ermini F, et al. Porphyromonas gingivalis in Alzheimer's disease brains: evidence for disease causation and treatment with small-molecule inhibitors. Sci Adv. 2019;5(1):eaau3333. https://doi.org/10.1126/sciadv.aau3333.
17. Aridi YS, Walker JL, Wright ORL. The association between the mediterranean dietary pattern and cognitive health: a systematic review. Nutrients. 2017;9(7):674. https://doi.org/10.3390/nu9070674.
18. Morris MC, Tangney CC, Wang Y, Sacks FM, Bennett DA, Aggarwal NT. MIND diet associated with reduced incidence of Alzheimer's disease. Alzheimers Dement. 2015;11(9):1007–14. https://doi.org/10.1016/j.jalz.2014.11.009.
19. Zhao Y, Jia M, Chen W, Liu Z. The neuroprotective effects of intermittent fasting on brain aging and neurodegenerative diseases via regulating mitochondrial function. Free Radic Biol Med. 2022;182:206–18. https://doi.org/10.1016/j.freeradbiomed.2022.02.021.
20. Oberlander C. A multi-domain approach to prevention and reversal of cognitive decline. Sci J Lander Coll Arts Sci. 2018;11(2). https://touroscholar.touro.edu/sjlcas/vol11/iss2/9.
21. Newton W, McManus A. Consumption of fish and Alzheimer's disease. J Nutr Health Aging. 2011;15(7):551–4552. https://doi.org/10.1007/s12603-011-0065-x.
22. Wu S, Ding Y, Wu F, Li R, Hou J, Mao P. Omega-3 fatty acids intake and risks of dementia and Alzheimer's disease: a meta-analysis. Neurosci Biobehav Rev. 2015;48:1–9. https://doi.org/10.1016/j.neubiorev.2014.11.008.
23. Simopoulos AP. Omega-3 fatty acids in inflammation and autoimmune diseases. J Am Coll Nutr. 2002;21(6):495–505. https://doi.org/10.1080/07315724.2002.10719248.
24. Smith PJ, Blumenthal JA, Hoffman BM, et al. Aerobic exercise and neurocognitive performance: a meta-analytic review of randomized controlled trials. Psychosom Med. 2010;72(3):239–52. https://doi.org/10.1097/PSY.0b013e3181d14633.
25. Ebrahimi K, Majdi A, Baghaiee B, Hosseini SH, Sadigh-Eteghad S. Physical activity and beta-amyloid pathology in Alzheimer's disease: a sound mind in a sound body. EXCLI J. 2017;16:959–72. https://doi.org/10.17179/excli2017-475.
26. Memme JM, Erlich AT, Phukan G, Hood DA. Exercise and mitochondrial health. J Physiol. 2021;599(3):803–17. https://doi.org/10.1113/JP278853.

Sleep in the Aging Brain

3

Swathi Charya, Yaminee Deepika Nandamuru,
and Lynn Kataria

Key Points

1. Sleep architecture changes with age and a good history are important to identify comorbid sleep disorders and optimize treatment and quality of life.
2. Common sleep disorders include insomnia, sleep-disordered breathing, rapid eye movement (REM) sleep behavior disorder, circadian rhythm sleep-wake disorders, and restless legs syndrome.
3. There is a bidirectional relationship between sleep and cognitive disorders.
4. The changes in sleep architecture, circadian rhythm shifts, increased presence of medical and psychiatric conditions, and polypharmacy are all contributing influences to the way sleep is affected in the elderly and common sleep disorders found in this population.

3.1 Introduction

Sleep is a quintessential part of life, vital to both physical and cognitive health, and a sense of well-being. The nature of sleep changes with aging. Aging has been associated with increased fragmentation of sleep, reduced sleep duration, and less deep sleep (slow wave sleep) [1]. Several factors can lead to sleep disturbances in advanced age, such as one or combinations of the following: medications, environmental changes, medical conditions, social factors, and mental health [1].

S. Charya · Y. D. Nandamuru · L. Kataria (✉)
Sleep Medicine Section, VA Medical Center Department of Neurology,
Washington, DC, USA

Department of Neurology and Rehabilitation Medicine, George Washington University
School of Medicine, Washington, DC, USA
e-mail: Lynn.Kataria@va.gov

E. L. Cobbs, C. P. Prather (eds.), *Diseases of the Mind*, Topics in Geriatric Care,
https://doi.org/10.1007/978-981-97-5995-8_3

Recognizing the impact of these factors and providing sleep strategies can have a positive impact on the quality of life with aging.

3.2 Sleep Architecture

The architecture of sleep displays a shift with age. Deficits in slow-wave sleep have been possibly linked to a decline in cognitive function [2]. Furthermore, there seems to be an increase in the number of awakenings and time spent awake at night. This is coupled with increase sleep latency and time to fall back asleep after nocturnal awakenings as well. Because of this increased fragmentation of sleep, naps are more common in older adults [1]. The amount of deep sleep was found to be reduced to 3.4% during midlife and advanced age compared to 18.9% during early adulthood [3]. Slow-wave sleep is characterized by large amplitude EEG waveforms, which require large numbers of healthy neurons for production. With the aging process, there is a decrease in the number of healthy neurons. Subsequently, there is a decrease in the amount of slow-wave sleep EEG generators rather than a decreased need for slow-wave sleep in the elderly population [4].

Because of the shallow nature of sleep in older adults, there may be less restful sleep, which can lead to a decreased sense of well-being and a decline in cognitive health. Sleep is governed by the circadian rhythm system and homeostatic mechanisms to balance sleep/wake cycles and stages of sleep. In addition to the decreased amount of slow-wave sleep, there are also changes to circadian rhythms. As one ages, the suprachiasmatic nucleus tends to deteriorate, leading to altered functioning of the circadian system and decreased responsiveness to external cues [5].

3.3 Sleep Disorders

Common ranges of sleep disorders found in older adults include insomnia, sleep-disordered breathing, restless legs syndrome (RLS), periodic limb movements of sleep, and rapid eye movement behavior disorder, to name a few. Older adults are at increased risk for sleep disorders due to underlying medical and psychiatric conditions, medication use, changes in sleep architecture, and a combination of these factors [5]. Recent studies have shown that disturbances in sleep can precede depression but can also lead to an increased overall risk of depression as well as dementia [6]. Insomnia and sleep disordered breathing have been found to be risk factors for Alzheimer's dementia [6]. It is paramount to have a good sleep history to arrive 1 at the correct diagnosis and tailor treatment (Table 3.1).

Table 3.1 Patient questionnaire for sleep history

Patient questionnaire
Bedtimes and waketimes
Number of awakenings and able to go back to sleep or not
Do they feel refreshed in the mornings
Snoring
Daytime sleepiness and napping
Environmental factors—TV/devices, external sounds, lights, and pets
Pain symptoms during sleep
GI symptoms during sleep (GERD)
Nasal congestion or coughing during sleep
Dreaming and dream enactment
Restless legs symptoms—Uncomfortable sensation in legs at night while resting
Tobacco, alcohol, illicit drug use
Exercise
Diet
Caffeine intake
Occupation—Shift worker or prior shift work
Medical disorders and medications that may contribute to disrupted sleep

3.4 Sleep-Disordered Breathing

Obstructive sleep apnea (OSA) is a common sleep disorder of older adults and can present differently compared to younger individuals. There is a weaker association with obesity and a stronger association with worsening of the upper airway anatomy as risk factors for sleep apnea in the older population [7]. Weakening of muscle tone leads to increased airway collapse in older adults [7]. The common presentation of snoring, witnessed apneas, and nocturia does not necessarily occur in older individuals, as symptoms can be more masked [8]. Increased associations with cognitive impairment, falls, stroke, nocturnal hypertension, and mortality have been found with obstructive sleep apnea in the older adult population [4]. Sleep-disordered breathing is associated with deficits in executive and psychomotor function, memory decline, as well as increased morbidity and mortality. Thus, treatment is recommended regardless of severity [4]. Sleep disorders are also more common in institutionalized patients, and the severity of sleep-disordered breathing was found to be higher in those with dementia [9]. One of the more common treatments for sleep apnea is continuous positive airway pressure (CPAP), which has shown benefits in older adults with respect to cardiovascular mortality [10], though adherence to CPAP can be challenging.

3.5 Insomnia

Insomnia is a common sleep disorder found in older adults. Sleep is more likely to be disrupted by external factors (such as light and sound) than sleep in younger individuals. Older adults have more complaints about their sleep, including frequent disturbances, frequent awakenings, increased sleep latency, and excessive daytime sleepiness [4]. Difficulty with initiation or maintenance of sleep coupled with daytime sleepiness defines insomnia. Older adults commonly experience chronic pain and polypharmacy, which can lead to or further worsen symptoms of insomnia [6]. Persistent insomnia can increase the risk of depression, particularly in women [9]. Non-pharmacologic treatment strategies should be considered first, given the adverse effects of medications. Cognitive behavioral therapy for insomnia (CBTi) is the first line of treatment [11], and brief behavioral interventions have proven effective in advanced-age populations [12].

3.6 Circadian Rhythm Sleep Disorders

With aging, the suprachiasmatic nucleus tends to deteriorate, leading to altered functioning of the circadian rhythm system and decreased responsiveness to external cues [5]. The circadian rhythm changes lead to an advanced phase cycle with earlier sleep times and wake times [13], where older adults tend to fall asleep earlier and wake up earlier in the day due to an advance of the rhythms of core body temperature and melatonin secretion.

In addition to the age-related reduction of sleep from the circadian rhythm mechanism, there is also a decreased homeostatic pressure for sleep in individuals [14]. As such, persons with irregular sleep wake rhythm disorder often experience daytime sleepiness and difficulties aligning their sleep times with those of societal norms [15].

3.7 Other Common Sleep Disorders

The risk for Restless Legs Syndrome (RLS) increases over the age of 40, and RLS constitutes a common sleep disorder in older persons. It is around two times more common in women than it is in men, and many of these patients have coexisting periodic limb movements [5]. The worsening symptoms and severity of RLS in the older patient population have been linked to diminished quality of life, including daily functioning and sense of well-being [8]. Rapid eye movement behavior (REM) disorder is a sleep disorder that is found mostly in older men. It has been linked to narcolepsy and other degenerative neurological disorders such as Parkinson's disease, Lewy body dementia, as well as multiple system atrophy [5]. Symptoms can include daytime sleepiness associated with acting out dreams or nightmares, as seen by violent behavior in sleep or falling out of bed. Melatonin is often preferred as an initial treatment over clonazepam due to its more favorable side effect profile and has been linked to a decrease in muscle tonicity during REM sleep [16].

3.8 Expected Changes in Sleep Related to Cognitive and Movement Disorders

In addition to sleep-related changes in the normal aging adult, there are many disorders that contribute to poor sleep, including cognitive disorders. The effects of sleep on cognition should also be noted, creating a bidirectional relationship between these disorders and sleep.

3.9 Alzheimer's Disease

Alzheimer's Disease is marked by a progressive decline in memory, specifically in episodic memory. Persons with dementia often have issues with sleep, including sundowning (a confusional state occurring in the late afternoon and lasting into the night) and nighttime wakefulness [17]. The effects of sleep disturbance can be related to worsening cognition [18]. Persons with dementia are at higher risk for obstructive sleep apnea, REM-related behavior disorders, and insomnia. Sleep changes are similar to those of the rest of the older adult population but are more severe. Sleep studies have shown higher fragmentations, decreased circadian amplitude, and phase shifts [19]. The exception to this is in REM sleep, which may be related to the neurophysiology of Alzheimer's. For example, the dysfunction of acetylcholine affects sleep-related disorders in this population. Furthermore, the pathophysiology of OSA may also be linked to the development of Alzheimer's disease, further potentiating the bidirectional relationship between sleep and dementia [20].

When considering diagnostic and treatment options, one must consider the utility of sleep studies and CPAP. Patients with dementia have more difficulty with adherence to sleep studies given electrodes and unfamiliar settings. Treatment options may also be limited as patients with more neuropsychiatric manifestations may not be able to tolerate CPAP, which is the mainstay of treatment for obstructive sleep apnea [17]. In addition to pharmacological treatments, light therapy can help patients with Alzheimer's Dementia with circadian entrainment [21].

3.10 Parkinson's Disease and Lewy Body Dementia

Parkinson's disease can manifest with changes in sleep prior to physical exam findings. This patient population may have REM sleep behavior disorder, daytime sleepiness, insomnia, or restless legs syndrome [22]. The effects on sleep may be due to several factors including medications, the neurophysiology of Parkinson's, and the clinical manifestations of Parkinson's [23]. Although the exact physiological evidence of how Parkinson's affects sleep is unknown, some studies suggest the basal ganglia may help regulate the sleep-wake cycle, which may ultimately lead to the sleep disorders seen in Parkinson's [23]. Factors that contribute to sleep changes include the use of dopaminergic agents and brain stimulation treatment modalities. There are several pharmacological and non-pharmacological options in treating patients with Parkinson's related sleep disturbances. It is important to consider drug interactions with dopaminergic agents. Sleep hygiene and cognitive behavioral therapy are good options as a primary or adjunctive treatment [24].

3.11 Implications for Sleep in Pain Syndromes

The effects of pain contribute to disturbed sleep patterns, ranging from effects on sleep quality to sleep latency. Older adults may experience pain secondary to chronic medical and psychiatric illness, injuries secondary to falls or systemic disease. The relationship between sleep and pain is bidirectional [25]. Studies have shown sleep changes with pain include sleep latency, sleep fragmentation, lesser total sleep time, and decreased perception of restful sleep [25]. In persons living with dementia and pain, arousals and total time spent asleep were two measures that were lower than the general population in this age group [26]. Although depression can be a confounding factor, studies have shown pain related to hip osteoarthritis can affect sleep even when adjusted for depression on the WOMAC scoring scale [27]. Multiple sources can contribute to pain in the older population [26]. Controlling pain ameliorates sleep disorders such as insomnia. In a population which already exhibits a decrease in sleep quality due to age-related changes, every effort should be made to control pain symptoms for better quality of life.

3.12 Conclusion

In summary, several factors influence the changes in sleep that take place in advanced age. This patient population is also more prone to health issues, including renal, cardiovascular, neurodegenerative disease, and respiratory disorders that can contribute to poor sleep [4]. Mental health disorders, including anxiety and depression, also play a significant role. Advanced-age patients with depression are more likely to report a coexisting sleep disturbance [8]. Sleep is a pillar for various aspects of health, including physical, cognitive, and mental health, as well as an underlying sense of well-being. It is important to distinguish the physiologic changes of healthy aging from the pathologic signs of common sleep disorders to provide effective treatment and improve quality of life.

References

1. Li J, Vitiello MV, Gooneratne NS. Sleep in normal aging. Sleep Med Clin. 2018;13(1):1–11.
2. Ancoli-Israel S, Ayalon L, Salzman C. Sleep in the elderly: normal variations and common sleep disorders. Harv Rev Psychiatry. 2008;16(5):279–86.
3. Van Cauter E, Leproult R, Plat L. Age-related changes in slow wave sleep and REM sleep and relationship with growth hormone and cortisol levels in healthy men. JAMA. 2000;284(7):861–8.
4. Benca RM, Teodorescu M. Sleep physiology and disorders in aging and dementia. Handb Clin Neurol. 2019;167:477–93.
5. Roepke SK, Ancoli-Israel S. Sleep disorders in the elderly. Indian J Med Res. 2010;131:302–10.
6. Gulia KK, Kumar VM. Sleep disorders in the elderly: a growing challenge. Psychogeriatrics. 2018;18:155–65.
7. Sadaf M, Johnson A, Daw J, Hashmi A, Khawaja I. Breathing related sleep disorders in the elderly. Psychiatr Ann Thorofare. 2018;48(6):287–91.
8. Mc Carthy CE. Sleep disturbance, sleep disorders and co-morbidities in the care of the older person. Med Sci (Basel). 2021;9(2):31.
9. Neikrug AB, Ancoli-Israel S. Gerontology Basel. 2010;56(2):181–9.
10. Martinez-Garcia MA, Campos-Rodriguez F, Catalan-Serra P, et al. Cardiovascular mortality in obstructive sleep apnea in the elderly: role of long-term continuous positive airway pressure treatment: a prospective observational study. Am J Respir Crit Care Med. 2012;186:909–16.
11. Qaseem A, Kansagara D, Forciea MA, Cooke M, Denberg TD. Clinical Guidelines Committee of the American College of Physicians. Management of chronic insomnia disorder in adults: a clinical practice guideline from the American College of Physicians. Ann Intern Med. 2016;165(2):125–33.
12. Buysse DJ, Germain A, Moul DE, et al. Efficacy of brief behavioral treatment for chronic insomnia in older adults. Arch Intern Med. 2011;171(10):887–95.
13. Feinsilver SH. Normal and abnormal sleep in the elderly. Clin Geriatr Med. 2021;37(3):377–86.
14. Dijk D, Duffy J, Czeisler CJ. Contribution of circadian physiology and sleep homeostasis to age-related changes in human sleep. Chronobiol Int. 2000;17(3):285–311.
15. Oyegbile T, Videnovic A. Irregular sleep-wake rhythm disorder. Neurol Clin. 2019;37(3):553–61.
16. McGrane IR, Leung JG, St Louis EK, Boeve BF. Melatonin therapy for REM sleep behavior disorder: a critical review of evidence. Sleep Med. 2015;16(1):19–26.
17. Wennberg AMV, Wu MN, Rosenberg PB, Spira AP. Sleep disturbance, cognitive decline, and dementia: a review. Semin Neurol. 2017;37(4):395–406.
18. Peter-Derex L, Yammine P, Bastuji H, Croisile B. Sleep and Alzheimer's disease. Sleep Med Rev. 2015;19:29–38.
19. Leng Y, Musiek ES, Hu K, Cappuccio FP, Yaffe K. Association between circadian rhythms and neurodegenerative diseases. Lancet Neurol. 2019;18(3):307–18.
20. Cipriani G, Lucetti C, Danti S, Nuti A. Sleep disturbances and dementia. Psychogeriatrics. 2015;15(1):65–74.
21. Videnovic A, Lazar AS, Barker RA, Overeem S. 'The clocks that time us'—circadian rhythms in neurodegenerative disorders. Nat Rev Neurol. 2014;10(12):683–93.
22. Zhang Y, Ren R, Sanford LD, Yang L, Zhou J, Tan L, et al. Sleep in Parkinson's disease: a systematic review and meta-analysis of polysomnographic findings. Sleep Med Rev. 2020;51:101281.
23. Zahed H, Zuzuarregui JRP, Gilron R, Denison T, Starr PA, Little S. The neurophysiology of sleep in Parkinson's disease. Mov Disord. 2021;36(7):1526–42.
24. Taximaimaiti R, Luo X, Wang XP. Pharmacological and non-pharmacological treatments of sleep disorders in Parkinson's disease. Curr Neuropharmacol. 2021;19(12):2233–49.
25. Keilani M, Crevenna R, Dorner TE. Sleep quality in subjects suffering from chronic pain. Wien Klin Wochenschr. 2018;130:31–6.

26. Evans CD, Kovach CR. The association between physiological sources of pain and sleep quality in older adults with and without dementia. Res Gerontol Nurs. 2020;13(6):297–308.
27. Martinez R, Reddy N, Mulligan EP, Hynan LS, Wells J. Sleep quality and nocturnal pain in patients with hip osteoarthritis. Medicine. 2019;98(41):e17464.

Mood Syndromes in Aging

4

Michael Levy and Paul Rosenberg

Key Points

1. Mood disorders are more common in older adults with medical illness, disability, and functional losses.
2. Older adults with depression are at higher risk for suicide, particularly after experiencing health, social, or financial stressors.
3. Effective treatments for depressive disorders include pharmacotherapy, psychotherapy, and neuromodulation.

4.1 Depressive Disorders

Over a quarter of community-dwelling older adults report depressive symptoms, most commonly mild dysphoria, while a smaller subset of patients have major depressive disorder (MDD). Institutionalized patients have higher rates than their community-dwelling peers, with a prevalence rate of 20% MDD and another 20–25% suffering from minor depressive disorder. Approximately half of all older persons diagnosed with MDD have their initial episode after the age of 60 [1].

The relationship between depressive symptoms and medical illness is reciprocal, with strokes being a good example. Depression increases the risk of having a stroke by 45% and the risk of having stroke-related mortality by 25%, while up to 1/3 of patients who have a stroke develop post-stroke depression [2]. Many other chronic

M. Levy
CPL Michael J. Crescenz VA Medical Center City, Philadelphia, PA, USA
e-mail: michael.levy@va.gov

P. Rosenberg (✉)
Johns Hopkins University, Baltimore, MD, USA
e-mail: prosenb@jhmi.edu

E. L. Cobbs, C. P. Prather (eds.), *Diseases of the Mind*, Topics in Geriatric Care,
https://doi.org/10.1007/978-981-97-5995-8_4

27. Bettio L, Thacker JS, Hutton C, Christie BR. Modulation of synaptic plasticity by exercise. In: Yau SY, So KF, editors. International review of neurobiology, Exercise on brain health, vol. 147. Academic Press; 2019. p. 295–322. https://doi.org/10.1016/bs.irn.2019.07.002.
28. Alty J, Farrow M, Lawler K. Exercise and dementia prevention. Pract Neurol. 2020;20(3):234–40. https://doi.org/10.1136/practneurol-2019-002335.
29. Wayne PM, Walsh JN, Taylor-Piliae RE, et al. Effect of tai chi on cognitive performance in older adults: systematic review and meta-analysis. J Am Geriatr Soc. 2014;62(1):25–39. https://doi.org/10.1111/jgs.12611.
30. Wang F, Lee EKO, Wu T, et al. The effects of tai chi on depression, anxiety, and psychological well-being: a systematic review and meta-analysis. Int J Behav Med. 2014;21(4):605–17. https://doi.org/10.1007/s12529-013-9351-9.
31. Walsh S, Brayne CE. Does playing a musical instrument prevent dementia? Alzheimers Dement. 2021;17(S10):e049684. https://doi.org/10.1002/alz.049684.
32. Luders E, Cherbuin N, Gaser C. Estimating brain age using high-resolution pattern recognition: younger brains in long-term meditation practitioners. NeuroImage. 2016;134:508–13. https://doi.org/10.1016/j.neuroimage.2016.04.007.
33. Tang YY, Hölzel BK, Posner MI. The neuroscience of mindfulness meditation. Nat Rev Neurosci. 2015;16(4):213–25. https://doi.org/10.1038/nrn3916.
34. Paller KA, Creery JD, Florczak SM, et al. Benefits of mindfulness training for patients with progressive cognitive decline and their caregivers. Am J Alzheimers Dis Other Dement. 2015;30(3):257–67. https://doi.org/10.1177/1533317514545377.
35. Hashizume S, Nakano M, Kubota K, et al. Mindfulness intervention improves cognitive function in older adults by enhancing the level of miRNA-29c in neuron-derived extracellular vesicles. Sci Rep. 2021;11:21848. https://doi.org/10.1038/s41598-021-01318-y.
36. Koenig HG. Research on religion, spirituality, and mental health: a review. Can J Psychiatry. 2009;54(5):283–91. https://doi.org/10.1177/070674370905400502.
37. Windsor TD, Curtis RG, Luszcz MA. Sense of purpose as a psychological resource for aging well. Dev Psychol. 51(7):975. https://doi.org/10.1037/dev0000023.

illnesses are associated with depression, including cardiovascular disease, diabetes mellitus, and osteoporosis. Depression may hasten biological aging, as shown by epigenetic markers and shorter telomere lengths [3], and is associated with obesity, frailty, diabetes, and increased platelet activation, which may increase the risk of stroke or myocardial infarction [1].

Risk factors for late-life depression (LLD) include dysfunction in reward, salience, and cognitive control networks, which determine the intensity of mood, cognitive, and motoric symptoms. Other factors include genetics, endocrine dysfunction, psychological factors, systemic inflammation, vascular disease, and amyloid accumulation [4]. Depression is a polygenic disorder, with the gene SLC6A4, located on chromosome 17 and coding for the serotonin transporter gene most often implicated [5]. Adrenocortical dysfunction, as evidenced by increased cortisol levels related to chronic stress, has been implicated in LLD. Risk factors for LLD often start in middle age, such as hypertension, diabetes mellitus, amyloid disposition, and increased cerebrovascular disease [6]. Psychological aspects include personality attributes, such as hopelessness, neuroticism, feelings of abandonment, and catastrophizing events. Common stressors precipitating LLD include chronic pain, unemployment, divorce, widowhood, poverty, and social isolation. Depressed older adults have increased impairment in activities of daily living (ADLs) and mobility restrictions several years after their depression diagnosis [7].

Cognitive impairment is often associated with depressive symptoms in late life, and when the depression improves, the cognition often improves (termed "pseudodementia") but with an increased risk of developing subsequent dementia. Depression can be the prodrome of neurodegenerative diseases such as Alzheimer's disease [8]. A growing area of research has been related to mild behavioral impairment (MBI), which describes the emergence at >50 years old of sustained and impactful neuropsychiatric symptoms (NPS) as a precursor to cognitive decline and dementia [9].

The prognosis of LLD is similar to younger adults in the absence of comorbid medical illness or functional/cognitive impairment, and depressive episodes usually partially remit. Patients that develop MDD superimposed on persistent depressive disorder have a particularly poor prognosis, similar to having poor social support or significant functional limitations. Recurrent depressive episodes in late life tend to be associated with similar symptoms and duration to early life [10], and the average duration of untreated depressive episodes averages 9 months. More frequent episodes can create a "kindling" effect, where repeated episodes make patients more vulnerable to worse and recurrent symptoms. Factors that are associated with better outcomes in LLD include good social support, history of quick recovery from prior depressive episodes, family history of depression, female gender, extroverted personality, lack of substance abuse or other mental disorders, employment, and absence of major negative life events.

Adults aged 75 or older in the US had suicide rates of 19.1 per 100,000 in 2020. Older adults tend to use more lethal suicide methods, such as firearms, and they are more likely to die from an attempt. Suicide risk is increased by depression severity, social isolation, chronic pain [11], recent loss of loved ones, feelings of loneliness, and financial stressors. Suicide risk should be routinely evaluated in depressed persons. Older adults with a recent diagnosis of mild cognitive impairment or dementia are at a particularly increased risk of suicide. A large study of United States veterans showed an increased rate of suicide of 73% for patients with a recent MCI diagnosis and 44% for a recent dementia diagnosis [12]. Given this, it is important to get involved in supportive services soon after a diagnosis.

Diagnostic and Statistical Manual (DSM-5) defines several depressive disorders [13]:

1. Major Depressive Disorder (MDD): at least 2 weeks of depressed mood and/or lack of interest/pleasure (anhedonia) with at least four other symptoms, including problems with sleep, interests, feeling of guilt, energy, concentration, psychomotor restlessness or retardation, appetite, suicidal ideation, or passive death wish. Psychotic delusions are relatively common in late life, often related to thoughts of persecution or having an incurable illness.
2. Persistent Depressive Disorder (PDD): depressive symptoms for at least 2 years, during which patients are never without symptoms for more than 2 months at a time, and they do not meet the criteria for MDD. Patients with PDD often develop periodic episodes of MDD.
3. Minor/subsyndromal depression (coded under the DSM-5 "Other specified depressive disorder") at least 2 weeks of depressed affect and at least one other symptom of major depression.
4. Depression due to another medical condition: evidence of depression due to the direct pathophysiologic consequences of a medical condition, common in post-myocardial infarctions and strokes, Parkinson's disease, and cancer.
5. Adjustment disorder with depressed mood: exhibition of a maladaptive reaction to an identifiable stressor within 3 months and symptoms are greater than expected levels.

History includes duration and severity of current episode, history of previous episodes, history of current or prior alcohol or illicit drug abuse, response to previous therapeutic interventions, family history of depression, assessing for cognitive status with a Montreal Objective Cognitive Assessment (MOCA) or Mini Mental Status Examination (MMSE), and a physical examination. Laboratory tests include a thyroid panel, complete blood count to evaluate for anemia, B12, folate, and complete metabolic panel to evaluate for vitamin deficiencies, electrolyte disturbances, kidney/hepatic function, and polysomnography if concerns for obstructive sleep apnea. There are no biological markers available to confirm the diagnosis of depression in clinical practice. An EKG should be obtained to evaluate for cardiac abnormalities and to assess for QTc prolongation. Depression symptom checklists are useful in determining the severity of illness, determining patient needs, and tracking symptom changes.

Treatment includes pharmacotherapy, neuromodulation, and psychotherapy [14] (Table 4.1). Selective serotonin reuptake inhibitors (SSRIs) are usually first-line due to their safety profile, low anticholinergic burden, and low propensity to cause

Table 4.1 Medications to treat depression in older adults

Class	Medications	Special comments
Selective serotonin reuptake inhibitors (SSRIs)	Fluoxetine, Fluvoxamine, Paroxetine, Sertraline, Citalopram, Escitalopram	Sexual dysfunction, GI distress, bleeding risk, dizziness, insomnia, mild weight gain, QT prolongation (citalopram).
Selective norepinephrine reuptake inhibitors (SNRIs)	Venlafaxine, Duloxetine, Desvenlafaxine	Also effective for chronic neuropathic pain. Similar side effect profile to SSRI's, less associated with weight gain. Can increase blood pressure.
Serotonin modulators	Vilazodone, Vortioxetine, Trazodone	Less associated with sexual dysfunction. Some evidence Vortioxetine associated with improved cognition.
Dopamine reuptake inhibitors	Bupropion	Good for smoking cessation and ADHD. Weight loss, tachycardia.
Tricyclic antidepressants (TCAs)	Amitriptyline, Clomipramine, Desipramine, Doxepin, Imipramine, Nortriptyline, Amoxapine, Protriptyline, Trimipramine	– Less frequently used, given significant anticholinergic side effects and cardiac toxicity in overdose. – Nortriptyline is the one most often used in geriatric depression, given the largest therapeutic window. – Low dose doxepin of 3–6 mg FDA approved and effective for insomnia with relatively safe side effect profile.
Monoamine oxidase inhibitors (MAOIs)	Tranylcypromine, Phenelzine, Selegiline, Isocarboxazid	– Significant drug–drug interactions that increase the risk of developing serotonin syndrome. – Use necessitates dietary restrictions to prevent hypertensive crisis.
Alpha 2 antagonist	Mirtazapine	Sedation, weight gain through increased appetite.

orthostasis or sedation. Five SSRIs are FDA approved for depression. Escitalopram and sertraline are usual choices, as they have relatively benign drug interactions and minimal QTc prolongation. Common side effects from SSRIs include nausea, sleep disturbances, activation, decreased libido, and weight gain. Serotonin/norepinephrine reuptake inhibitors (SNRIs) may be helpful for neuropathic pain and have less effect on libido and weight gain. Common side effects with SNRIs include hypertension and dizziness, particularly with venlafaxine. Among tricyclic antidepressants, nortriptyline is most used, given its relatively favorable therapeutic window and low anticholinergic burden. Psychostimulants can be beneficial in LLD, particularly if the patient is suffering from anergia or apathy. Other options include mirtazapine, bupropion, vortioxetine, vilazodone, and atypical antipsychotics.

Esketamine was recently approved by the FDA as an augmenting agent for treatment-resistant depression and has been shown to be relatively safe and effective in older adults. Pharmacotherapy starts low and goes slow. Older adults are more likely to experience adverse effects such as serotonin syndrome, hyponatremia due to syndrome of inappropriate antidiuretic hormone secretion (SIADH), and anticholinergic effects such as constipation, sedation, and blurry vision.

Neuromodulation for LLD includes electroconvulsive therapy (ECT) and transcranial magnetic stimulation (TMS). ECT has been considered the gold standard for severe or treatment-refractory LLD and should be considered in patients with severe depression who have not responded to pharmacotherapy or who have life-threatening consequences of LLD such as suicidality or severe weight loss. ECT leads to more rapid improvement in LLD than medication as well as lower rates of rehospitalization and suicide up to 1 year out from treatment [15, 16]. It is generally safe to use for patients with comorbid neurological, pulmonary, or cardiac conditions. Most common side effects include headache and temporary amnesia, both retrograde and anterograde. Long-term cognitive changes are rare, and cognition often improves after completion of an ECT course [17]. The number of ECT sessions needed for response and remission of symptoms varies, typically between 6 and 12 sessions, performed 3 days/week. TMS is FDA approved for depression and is effective in older adults. Magnets are used to stimulate critical cortical pathways in depression, such as the dorsolateral prefrontal cortex. It requires a series of sessions, typically 5 days/week for 4–6 weeks.

Psychotherapy is effective in LLD, with or without pharmacotherapy, and the two have synergistic effects [18]. Cognitive behavioral therapy (CBT) aims to change behaviors through restructuring negative automatic thoughts. The benefits of CBT include being directive and time-limited, usually 10–25 sessions. Problem-solving therapy (PST) is a variant of CBT that is particularly effective in patients with executive dysfunction.

4.2 Bipolar and Related Disorders

Bipolar disorder is an often severe, relapsing and remitting cycling illness that affects the ability to regulate moods, which can be manic, hypomanic, or depressed. Disorders include bipolar 1 and 2 disorders, substance-induced bipolar disorder, and cyclothymia [13]. The prevalence of bipolar disorder decreases with age, although it is a frequent cause of inpatient psychiatric admissions in late life [10, 19]. The mortality rate for patients with bipolar disorder is increased when compared to the general population or those with unipolar depression. Older age bipolar disorder (OABD) occurs in patients 60 years of age and older, comprises about 25% of all patients with bipolar disorder and is expected to grow over the next decade. About 5–10% of patients with bipolar disorder will be over 50 years old at the time of having their first manic or hypomanic episode, termed late-onset bipolar disorder (LOBD). LOBD is associated with cerebrovascular disease, decreased rates of psychotic features, and increased rates of recurrence [20]. Overall relapse rates in symptoms lead to psychiatric hospitalizations decrease with age, possibly due to attenuation of symptom severity. OABD is associated with decreased gray matter volume and white matter hyperintensities, which are thought to be evidence of vascular disease, and with medical comorbidities and death on average 10 years earlier compared to the general population. Cognitive dysfunction is prevalent, particularly in LOBD, suggesting that different mechanisms may underlie the pathophysiology of early and LOBD. Depressive episodes are more common than manic or hypomanic episodes in late life and are often the initial mood episode, often with 10–20 years between the initial depressive episode and the first manic episode.

1. Bipolar 1 disorder: at least 1 week of mania where the mood is euphoric, expansive, or irritable and be accompanied by at least three of the following seven symptoms: the decreased need for sleep, racing thoughts, pressured speech, grandiosity, increase in goal-directed activity/psychomotor agitation, distractible, and/or engaging in risk-taking activities/behaviors. Patients do not need to have experienced a depressive illness, but many will.
2. Bipolar 2 disorder: the patient must experience hypomanic symptoms for at least 4 days and have a history of major depressive disorder. Symptoms do not interfere with social or occupational functioning to any significant degree.
3. Cyclothymic disorder: at least 2 years of numerous periods of hypomanic and depressive symptoms that do not meet the criteria for hypomanic episodes or MDD. Many patients will develop bipolar 1 or 2 disorders in their lifetime.

Lithium and valproic acid are the preferred choices for monotherapy for OAPD [21, 22]. Other treatments include lamotrigine, which is particularly effective at treating and preventing depressive episodes, and atypical antipsychotics.

Lithium Therapeutic doses often need to be lower in older patients, given decreased renal clearance and longer half-life. Commonly prescribed medications can have strong effects on lithium levels. ACE-inhibitors, thiazide diuretics, and nonsteroidal anti-inflammatory drugs increase lithium levels, while caffeine lowers lithium levels. Lithium levels for maintenance therapy should be 0.4–0.8 in patients 60–79 and 0.4–0.7 in patients over 80. Lithium can worsen thyroid and renal dysfunction. Adverse effects include cognitive impairment, ataxia, weight gain, and tremor. Assessment should include lithium level, creatinine, GFR, BUN, TSH, fasting glucose, lipids, calcium, a complete blood count, cognitive screening with a MMSE or MOCA, and physical examination looking at gait and assessing for tremor. Older adults are more susceptible to lithium toxicity with delirium, tremors, ataxia, nausea, vomiting, and inability to sustain and shift attention. Patients with these symptoms should be emergently evaluated and treated.

Valproic Acid (Depakote) Therapeutic doses will often be lower in older patients. Therapeutic blood levels range from 50 to 120. Older adults have an increased free fraction (active) portion of the drug, and total drug levels may underrepresent actual levels. Aspirin can increase the free fraction of the drug. Depakote increases the unbound fraction of warfarin. The drug is available in sprinkle and liquid formulations, which can benefit patients with difficulty swallowing. Common side effects include nausea, somnolence, and weight gain.

References

1. Steffens DC, Blazer DG, Thakur ME. The American Psychiatric Publishing Textbook of Geriatric Psychiatry. 5th ed. American Psychiatric Publishing; 2015.
2. Daskalopoulou M, et al. Depression as a risk factor for the initial presentation of twelve cardiac, cerebrovascular, and peripheral arterial diseases: data linkage study of 1.9 million women and men. PLoS One. 2016;11:e0153838. https://doi.org/10.1371/journal.pone.0153838.
3. Han LKM, et al. Epigenetic aging in major depressive disorder. Am J Psychiatry. 2018;175:774–82. https://doi.org/10.1176/appi.ajp.2018.17060595.
4. Alexopoulos GS. Mechanisms and treatment of late-life depression. Transl Psychiatry. 2019;9(1):188. https://doi.org/10.1038/s41398-019-0514-6.
5. Lam D, Ancelin ML, Ritchie K, et al. Genotype-dependent associations between serotonin transporter gene (*SLC6A4*) DNA methylation and late-life depression. BMC Psychiatry. 2018;18:282. https://doi.org/10.1186/s12888-018-1850-4.
6. Williamson W, et al. Association of cardiovascular risk factors with MRI indices of cerebrovascular structure and function and white matter hyperintensities in young adults. JAMA. 2018;320:665–73. https://doi.org/10.1001/jama.2018.11498.
7. Coventry PA, McMillan D, Clegg A, et al. Frailty and depression predict instrumental activities of daily living in older adults: a population-based longitudinal study using the CARE75+ cohort. PLoS One. 2020;15(12):e0243972. https://doi.org/10.1371/journal.pone.0243972.
8. Singh-Manoux A, Dugravot A, Fournier A, et al. Trajectories of depressive symptoms before diagnosis of dementia: a 28-year follow-up study. JAMA Psychiatry. 2017;74(7):712–8. https://doi.org/10.1001/jamapsychiatry.2017.0660.
9. Lyketsos CG. Neuropsychiatric symptoms in dementia: overview and measurement challenges. J Prev Alzheimers Dis. 2015;2(3):155–6. https://doi.org/10.14283/jpad.2015.60.
10. Haigh EAP, Bogucki OE, Sigmon ST, et al. Depression among older adults: a 20-year update on five common myths and misconceptions. Am J Geriatr Psychiatry. 2018;26(1):107–22. https://doi.org/10.1016/j.jagp.2017.06.011.
11. Choi NG, DiNitto DM, Marti CN, et al. Suicide means among decedents aged 50+ years, 2005-2014: trends and associations with sociodemographic and precipitating factors. Am J Geriatr Psychiatry. 2017;25(12):1404–14. https://doi.org/10.1016/j.jagp.2017.06.001.
12. Günak MM, Barnes DE, Yaffe K, et al. Risk of suicide attempt in patients with recent diagnosis of mild cognitive impairment or dementia. JAMA Psychiatry. 2021;78(6):659–66. https://doi.org/10.1001/jamapsychiatry.2021.0150.
13. American Psychiatric Association. Diagnostic and statistical manual of mental disorders. 5th ed; 2013. https://doi.org/10.1176/appi.books.9780890425596.
14. Kok RM, Reynolds CF 3rd. Management of depression in older adults: a review. JAMA. 2017;317(20):2114–22. https://doi.org/10.1001/jama.2017.5706.
15. van Rooij SJH, Riva-Posse P, McDonald WM. The efficacy and safety of neuromodulation treatments in late-life depression. Curr Treat Options Psychiatry. 2020;7(3):337–48. https://doi.org/10.1007/s40501-020-00216-w.
16. Rhebergen D, et al. Older age is associated with rapid remission of depression after electroconvulsive therapy: a latent class growth analysis. Am J Geriatr Psychiatry. 2015;23(3):274–82.

17. Kellner CH, Husain MM, Knapp RG, et al. A novel strategy for continuation ECT in geriatric depression: phase 2 of the PRIDE study. Am J Psychiatry. 2016;173(11):1110–8. https://doi.org/10.1176/appi.ajp.2016.16010118.
18. Raue PJ, McGovern AR, Kiosses DN, et al. Advances in psychotherapy for depressed older adults. Curr Psychiatry Rep. 2017;19(9):57. https://doi.org/10.1007/s11920-017-0812-8.
19. Dols A, Kessing LV, Strejilevich SA, et al. Do current national and international guidelines have specific recommendations for older adults with bipolar disorder? A brief report. Int J Geriatr Psychiatry. 2016;31(12):1295–300. https://doi.org/10.1002/gps.4534.
20. Sajatovic M, Strejilevich SA, Gildengers AG, et al. A report on older-age bipolar disorder from the International Society for Bipolar Disorders Task Force. Bipolar Disord. 2015;17(7):689–704. https://doi.org/10.1111/bdi.12331.
21. Shulman KI, Almeida OP, Herrmann N, et al. Delphi survey of maintenance lithium treatment in older adults with bipolar disorder: an ISBD task force report. Bipolar Disord. 2019;21(2):117–23. https://doi.org/10.1111/bdi.12714.
22. Young RC, Mulsant BH, Sajatovic M, et al. GERI-BD: a randomized double-blind controlled trial of lithium and divalproex in the treatment of mania in older patients with bipolar disorder. Am J Psychiatry. 2017;174(11):1086–93. https://doi.org/10.1176/appi.ajp.2017.15050657.

Stroke and Implications for Brain Health

5

Benny Kim, Sabena Passarello, and Zurab Nadareishvili

Key Points

1. Poststroke cognitive impairment and dementia (PSCID) occurs in 10–30% of patients with stroke and is associated with age, education, stroke severity, and stroke recurrence.
2. No intervention exists to prevent PSCID. PSCID carries a higher risk of stroke recurrence and death.
3. Poststroke depression (PSD) is a common complication associated with stroke and occurs in 31% of patients.
4. Possible treatment modalities for PSD include SSRIs and SNRIs, as well as cognitive behavioral therapy and exercise.

5.1 Implications of Stroke on Cognitive Impairment

Cerebrovascular disease-related vascular cognitive impairment is the second most common cause of dementia after Alzheimer's disease [1]. Poststroke cognitive impairment and dementia (PSCID), on the other hand, is one of the most common causes of vascular cognitive impairment. In a large meta-analysis, PSCID rates ranged from 7.4% in population-based studies of first-ever stroke in which prestroke dementia was excluded to 41.3% in hospital-based studies of recurrent stroke in which prestroke dementia was included [2]. Approximately 10% of patients will

B. Kim · S. Passarello · Z. Nadareishvili (✉)
Department of Neurology and Rehabilitation Medicine, The George Washington University School of Medicine and Health Sciences, Washington, DC, USA

Comprehensive Stroke Center, VHC Health, Arlington, VA, USA
e-mail: bekim@mfa.gwu.edu; spassarello@mfa.gwu.edu; znadareishvili@mfa.gwu.edu

E. L. Cobbs, C. P. Prather (eds.), *Diseases of the Mind*, Topics in Geriatric Care,
https://doi.org/10.1007/978-981-97-5995-8_5

develop dementia after the first stroke, and more than 33% have dementia after recurrent stroke [2].

The risk of PSCID largely depends on stroke severity [3]. The incidence of PSCID at 1 year was 34.4% in patients with severe stroke, 8.2% in those with minor stroke, and 5.2% in those with transient ischemic attack [3]. Five-year risk of dementia, in addition to stroke severity, was associated with age, previous stroke, dysphasia, baseline cognition, low education, premorbid dependency, leukoaraiosis, and diabetes [3].

Although small vessel disease-related stroke volume is low, lacunar stroke carries the same risk of PSCID as other subtypes of stroke with larger volume [4]. Subgroup analysis of the SPS-3 (Stroke Prevention in Small Subcortical Stroke) trial showed that 47% of patients with lacunar stroke had mild cognitive impairment at the time of randomization at a median of 60 days after the initial stroke [5]. Older age, male sex, less education, poststroke disability, and impaired activities of daily living were independently associated with PSCID [5].

Older age is associated with faster cognitive decline after stroke. In the REGARDS (Reasons for Geographic and Racial Differences in Stroke) study, each 1-year increase in baseline age was associated with a 17% higher risk of cognitive impairment per year of follow-up [6].

Although traditional stroke risk factors, including hypertension, diabetes, and hyperlipidemia, are implicated in the pathophysiology of PSCID, there is limited evidence from clinical trials that risk factor management may prevent PSCID. Blood pressure (BP) lowering therapy had no effect on PSCID prevention in two clinical trials [7, 8]. On the other hand, another two clinical trials showed a modest effect of BP-lowering therapy on PSCID prevention [9, 10]. However, the quality of evidence is insufficient to recommend intensive BP lowering solely for the prevention of PSCID. Similar to BP management, neither cholesterol-lowering therapy nor antidiabetic treatment for insulin resistance failed to prevent PSCID [11, 12].

PSCID is associated with significant disability, dependency, increased morbidity, and mortality. In a subgroup analysis of the SPS3 trial that enrolled a cohort of nondisabled and nondemented patients with lacunar stroke, poststroke global cognitive impairment was associated with an increased risk of all-cause mortality, while memory impairment was associated with an increased risk of recurrent stroke and death [13]. In another subgroup analysis of IRIS (Insulin Resistance Intervention in Stroke) trial including 3338 patients with stroke and insulin resistance, impairments in language and orientation were associated with 35–40% higher risk of recurrent stroke, while attention impairment was associated with 34% increase in all-cause mortality. In both studies, reported associations were independent of age, gender, race/ethnicity, education, BP and glucose control, clinical trial treatment allocation, cardiovascular disease and stroke history, smoking status, as well as stroke severity and disability, suggesting the involvement of different mechanisms rather than traditional stroke risk factors. One explanation might be the crosstalk between neurodegeneration and vascular pathologies, including cerebral amyloid angiopathy. In the SPS3 trial, patients with lobar microbleeds, which is one of the clinical phenotypes of cerebral amyloid angiopathy, had a higher risk of recurrent stroke compared to those without it [13].

5.2 Implications for Stroke on Depression

Poststroke depression (PSD) is an important psychological disorder that can impair the quality of life and functional recovery after a stroke. Some characteristic features include depressed mood, lack of interest in activities, poor appetite, sleep disturbances, and loss of energy [14]. Studies suggest that 31% of individuals recovering from stroke develop PSD in the first 5 years after the stroke [15]. Decreased rates of PSD have been found as time elapsed beyond the stroke incident, as rates were 25% between 2 and 5 years and 23% at 5 years after stroke [15].

Certain features of baseline stroke disability factor into the development of PSD; for instance, stroke severity, determined by higher NIH Stroke Scale (NIHSS) scores, has been associated with an increased risk of PSD within the first year of recovery after stroke [16]. Aphasia after stroke was associated with higher rates of PSD [17]. In addition, symptoms of PSD were higher in individuals with higher (worse) scores on the Modified Rankin Scale (mRS), a tool used to identify the level of functional independence [16]. Women have a higher risk of PSD than men [18]. Older individuals, in particular those above the age of 70, were found to have higher rates of PSD [16]. Another risk factor for PSD is a history of depression or anxiety prior to stroke [16, 19].

Many tools can be utilized to diagnose PSD. The Center of Epidemiological Studies-Depression Scale (CESD), the Hamilton Depression Rating Scale (HDRS), and the Patient Health Questionnaire (PHQ)-9 have been identified as optimal for PSD diagnosis [20].

A meta-analysis reviewed imaging studies for stroke and identified frontal/anterior, subcortical, and basal ganglia lesions that were frequently associated with PSD [21]. This study found 54% higher odds of PSD after frontal stroke [21]. These findings were evident after the acute phase of stroke, described as 15 days to 6 months [21]. Other imaging findings included cerebral atrophy, white matter hyperintensities, microbleeds, large infarct volume, and a large number of infarcts [21]. Laterality of stroke was not found to have a significant effect on the development of PSD [21].

Strokes precipitate abnormal intrinsic functional connectivity in networks supporting the experience and regulation of emotions, notably the cognitive control network [22]. Weaker connectivity in such areas, like the dorsolateral prefrontal cortex and the supramarginal gyrus, has been linked to higher rates of depression [22]. Strokes have also been shown to lead to depression due to changes in neurotransmitter dysregulation, changes in cortisol levels, and increased pro-inflammatory cytokines [22, 23]. While PSD leads to negative effects on brain pathways and overall brain health, it also contributes to an increased risk of all-cause mortality [23]. Some data suggest that PSD has an effect on stroke recurrence, as well, but no strong association has been established [23].

While treatment options are available for PSD, data suggests many individuals are untreated. The rate of treatment for PSD was 17.7% in 2004–2005 and 16.0% in 2016–2017 [24]. Successful treatment modalities for PSD include antidepressant medications, cognitive behavioral therapy, and exercise [14]. Among medications for PSD, selective serotonin reuptake inhibitors (SSRIs) and serotonin-norepinephrine reuptake inhibitors (SNRIs) have shown the greatest benefits [14]. The establishment of support structures for individuals with stroke is also helpful in stroke rehabilitation and depression management [17].

5.3 Prognostication for Brain Health After Stroke: Guidance for Clinicians and Families

Stroke sequellae range from death to disability to complete recovery. Predicting these outcomes is of importance to patients, families, and clinicians [25]. Prognostication can be difficult, and studies have demonstrated that clinicians have low accuracy in predicting stroke outcomes, even those with stroke expertise [26]. Only 1 in 6 (16.9%) clinicians accurately predicted death or disability at discharge after stroke in one study [27]. Most of the prognostic scales focus on predicting mortality or long-term disability. Prediction of cognitive functioning after stroke is an outcome that can be overlooked in both patients with severe physical disability and those deemed completely recovered [28].

A review of the quality of 10 better-known stroke scales described in the literature found that they often utilized similar input variables, and most had reasonable accuracy. These scales commonly measured patient demographics, comorbidity, initial stroke severity as measured by NIHSS, and prestroke functional status [25]. Five scales, Totaled Health Risks in Vascular Events Stroke (THRIVE); Acute Stroke Registry and Analysis of Lausanne (ASTRAL); Dense Artery, mRS, Age, Glucose, Onset-to-Treatment, and NIHSS (DRAGON); the iScore; Stroke Subtype, OCSP, Age, and Pre-stroke mRS (SOAR), have been validated by multiple independent studies, and the latter four had sufficient predictive ability to merit implementation into clinical practice [29–33]. Other scales require further research to confirm their prognostic value [25]. The ASTRAL and DRAGON scales were found to predict patient outcomes better than physicians, even those with stroke expertise [34]. The DRAGON scale incorporates an acute stroke neuroimaging characteristic (a hyperdense artery sign and/or early infarct signs on CT), in addition to the five other variables to predict functional outcomes 3 months poststroke in patients who received acute thrombolysis [25].

PSCID is common after stroke, and 10% of patients will develop new dementia soon after the first stroke, while 30% after recurrent stroke [3, 35]. Acute neuroimaging in stroke is primarily used to determine eligibility for receiving thrombolysis. However, certain imaging characteristics have been associated with an increased risk of developing PSCID. One meta-analysis reviewed 28 studies to identify neuroimaging features that were associated with developing PSCID [35]. The length of follow-up to assess for PSCID ranged from 3 months to 6 years poststroke in the trials reviewed, and some trials included patients with ischemic and hemorrhagic stroke [35]. The presence of cerebral atrophy, white matter lesions (WML), and preexisting stroke lesions on acute neuroimaging were associated with a two- to threefold increase in the risk of developing PSCID. In terms of developing cognitive impairment, only WML were associated with an increased risk after stroke [35].

Utilizing both neuroimaging and validated prognostic stroke scales allows the clinician to predict the gross functional outcome and risk of developing PSCID after stroke.

References

1. Prince M, Bryce R, Albanese E, Wimo A, Ribeiro W, Ferri CP. The global prevalence of dementia: a systematic review and meta-analysis. Alzheimers Dement. 2013;9(1):63–75. https://doi.org/10.1016/j.jalz.2012.11.007.
2. Pendlebury ST, Rothwell PM. Prevalence, incidence, and factors associated with pre-stroke and post-stroke dementia: a systematic review and meta-analysis. Lancet Neurol. 2009;8:1006–18. https://doi.org/10.1016/S1474-4422(09)70236-4.
3. Pendlebury ST, Rothwell PM. Incidence and prevalence of dementia associated with transient ischaemic attack and stroke: analysis of the population-based Oxford Vascular Study. Lancet Neurol. 2019;8:248–58. https://doi.org/10.1016/S1474-4422(18)30442-3.
4. Makin SD, Turpin S, Dennis MS, Wardlaw JM. Cognitive impairment after lacunar stroke: systematic review and meta-analysis of incidence, prevalence and comparison with other stroke subtypes. J Neurol Neurosurg Psychiatry. 2013;84(8):893–900. https://doi.org/10.1136/jnnp-2012-303645.
5. Jacova C, Pearce LA, Costello R, McClure LA, Holliday SL, Hart RG, et al. Cognitive impairment in lacunar strokes: the SPS3 trial. Ann Neurol. 2012;72(3):351–62. https://doi.org/10.1002/ana.23733.
6. Levine DA, Wadley VG, Langa KM, Unverzagt FW, Kabeto MU, Giordani B, Howard G, Howard VJ, Cushman M, Judd SE, et al. Risk factors for poststroke cognitive decline: the REGARDS Study (Reasons for Geographic and Racial Differences in Stroke). Stroke. 2018;49:987–94. https://doi.org/10.1161/STROKEAHA.117.018529.
7. Diener HC, Sacco RL, Yusuf S, Cotton D, Ounpuu S, Lawton WA, Palesch Y, Martin RH, Albers GW, Bath P, et al. Effects of aspirin plus extended-release dipyridamole versus clopidogrel and telmisartan on disability and cognitive function after recurrent stroke in patients with ischaemic stroke in the Prevention Regimen for Effectively Avoiding Second Strokes (PRoFESS) trial: a double-blind, active and placebo-controlled study. Lancet Neurol. 2008;7:875–84. https://doi.org/10.1016/S1474-4422(08)70198-4.
8. Pearce LA, McClure LA, Anderson DC, Jacova C, Sharma M, Hart RG, Benavente OR. Effects of long-term blood pressure lowering and dual antiplatelet treatment on cognitive function in patients with recent lacunar stroke: a secondary analysis from the SPS3 randomised trial. Lancet Neurol. 2014;13:1177–85. https://doi.org/10.1016/S1474-4422(14)70224-8.
9. Zheng H, Wang Y, Wang A, Li H, Wang D, Zhao X, Wang P, Shen H, Zuo L, Pan Y, et al. The efficacy and safety of nimodipine in acute ischemic stroke patients with mild cognitive impairment: a double-blind, randomized, placebo-controlled trial. Sci Bull. 2019;64:101–7. https://doi.org/10.1016/j.scib.2018.12.006.
10. PROGRESS Collaborative Group. Randomised trial of a perindopril-based blood-pressure lowering regimen among 6,105 individuals with previous stroke or transient ischaemic attack. Lancet. 2001;358:1033–41. https://doi.org/10.1016/S0140-6736(01)06178-5.
11. Hosomi N, Nagai Y, Kohriyama T, Ohtsuki T, Aoki S, Nezu T, Maruyama H, Sunami N, Yokota C, Kitagawa K, et al. The Japan Statin Treatment Against Recurrent Stroke (J-STARS): a mul-

ticenter, randomized, open-label, parallel-group study. EBioMedicine. 2015;2:1071–8. https://doi.org/10.1016/j.ebiom.2015.08.006.
12. Furie KL, Viscoli CM, Gorman M, Ford GA, Young LH, Inzucchi SE, Guarino PD, Lovejoy AM, Conwit R, Tanne D, Kernan WN. Effects of pioglitazone on cognitive function in patients with a recent ischaemic stroke or TIA: a report from the IRIS trial. J Neurol Neurosurg Psychiatry. 2018;89(1):21–7. https://doi.org/10.1136/jnnp-2017-316361.
13. Shoamanesh A, Pearce LA, Bazan C, Catanese L, McClure LA, Sharma M, et al. Microbleeds in the secondary prevention of small subcortical strokes trial: stroke, mortality, and treatment interactions. Ann Neurol. 2017;82(2):196–207. https://doi.org/10.1002/ana.24988.
14. Zhang S, Xu M, Liu Z, Feng J, Ma Y. Neuropsychiatric issues after stroke: clinical significance and therapeutic implications. World J Psychiatry. 2008;10(6):125–38. https://doi.org/10.5498/wjp.v10.i6.125.
15. Hackett M, Pickles K. Part 1: frequency of depression after stroke: an updated systematic review and meta-analysis of observational studies. Int J Stroke. 2014;9(8):1017–25. https://doi.org/10.1111/ijs.12357.
16. Almeida O, Hankey G, Ford A, Etherton-Beer C, Flicker L, Hackett M. Measures associated with early, late, and persistent clinically significant symptoms of depression 1 year after stroke in the AFFINITY trial. Neurology. 2022;98(10):e1021–30. https://doi.org/10.1212/WNL.0000000000200058.
17. Baker C, Worrall L, Rose M, Hudson K, Ryan B, O'Byrne L. A systematic review of rehabilitation interventions to prevent and treat depression in post-stroke aphasia. Disabil Rehabil. 2016;40(16):1870–92. https://doi.org/10.1080/09638288.2017.1315181.
18. Poynter B, Hon M, Diaz-Granados N, Kapral M, Grace S, Stewart D. Sex differences in the prevalanece of post-stroke depression: a systematic review. Psychosomatics. 2009;50(6):563–9. https://doi.org/10.1016/S0033-3182(09)70857-6.
19. Mayman N, Stein L, Erdman J, Kornspun A, Tuhrim S, Jette N, Dharmoon M. Risk and predictors of depression following acute ischemic stroke in the elderly. Neurology. 2021;96(17):e2184–91. https://doi.org/10.1212/WNL.0000000000011828.
20. Meader N, Moe-Byrne T, Llewellyn A, Mitchell A. Screening for poststroke major depression: a meta-analysis of diagnostic validity studies. J Neurol Neurosurg Psychiatry. 2014;85(2):198–206. https://doi.org/10.1136/jnnp-2012-304194.
21. Douven E, Köhler S, Rodriguez M, Staals J, Verhey F, Aalten P. Imaging markers of post-stroke depression and apathy: a systematic review and meta-analysis. Neuropsychol Rev. 2017;27:202–19. https://doi.org/10.1007/s11065-017-9356-2.
22. Jaywant A, DelPonte L, Kanellopoulos D, O'Dell M, Gunning F. The structural and functional neuroanatomy of post-stroke depression and executive dysfunction: a review of neuroimaging findings and implications for treatment. J Geriatr Psychiatry Neurol. 2020;35(1):3–11. https://doi.org/10.1177/0891988720968270.
23. Cai W, Muelller C, Li Y, Shen W, Stewart R. Post stroke depression and risk of stroke recurrence and mortality: a systematic review and meta-analysis. Ageing Res Rev. 2019;50:102–9. https://doi.org/10.1016/j.arr.2019.01.013.
24. Dong L, Mezuk B, Williams L, Lisabeth L. Trends in outpatient treatment for depression in survivors of stroke in the United States, 2004–2017. Neurology. 2022;98(22):e2258–67. https://doi.org/10.1212/WNL.0000000000200286.
25. Drozdowska BA, Singh S, Quinn TJ. Thinking about the future: a review of prognostic scales used in acute stroke. Front Neurol. 2019;10:274. https://doi.org/10.3389/fneur.2019.00274.
26. Gao MM, Wang J, Saposnik G. The art and science of stroke outcome prognostication. Stroke. 2020;51(5):1358–60. https://doi.org/10.1161/STROKEAHA.120.028980.
27. Saposnik G, Cote R, Mamdani M, Raptis S, Thorpe KE, Fang J, et al. JURaSSiC: accuracy of clinician vs risk score prediction of ischemic stroke outcomes. Neurology. 2013;81:448–55. https://doi.org/10.1212/WNL.0b013e31829d874e.
28. Sun JH, Tan L, Yu JT. Post-stroke cognitive impairment: epidemiology, mechanisms and management. Ann Transl Med. 2014;2(8):80. https://doi.org/10.3978/j.issn.2305-5839.2014.08.05.

29. Flint AC, Cullen SP, Faigeles BS, Rao VA. Predicting long-term outcome after endovascular stroke treatment: the totaled health risks in vascular events score. Am J Neuroradiol. 2010;31:1192–6. https://doi.org/10.3174/ajnr.A2050.
30. Ntaios G, Faouzi M, Ferrari J, Lang W, Vemmos K, Michel P. An integer-based score to predict functional outcome in acute ischemic stroke: the ASTRAL score. Neurology. 2012;78:1916–22. https://doi.org/10.1212/WNL.0b013e318259e221.
31. Strbian D, Meretoja A, Ahlhelm FJ, Pitkäniemi J, Lyrer P, Kaste M, et al. Predicting outcome of IV thrombolysis–treated ischemic stroke patients. The DRAGON score. Neurology. 2012;78:427–32. https://doi.org/10.1212/WNL.0b013e318245d2a9.
32. Saposnik G, Kapral MK, Liu Y, Hall R, O'Donnell M, Raptis S, et al. IScore: a risk score to predict death early after hospitalization for an acute ischemic stroke. Circulation. 2011;123:739–U172. https://doi.org/10.1161/CIRCULATIONAHA.110.983353.
33. Myint PK, Clark AB, Kwok CS, Davis J, Durairaj R, Dixit AK, et al. The SOAR (Stroke subtype, Oxford Community Stroke Project Classification, Age, prestroke modified Rankin) score strongly predicts early outcomes in acute stroke. Int J Stroke. 2014;9:278–83. https://doi.org/10.1111/ijs.12088.
34. Ntaios G, Gioulekas F, Papavasileiou V, Strbian D, Michel P. ASTRAL, DRAGON and SEDAN scores predict stroke outcome more accurately than physicians. Eur J Neurol. 2016;23:1651–7. https://doi.org/10.1111/ene.13100.
35. Ball EL, Sutherland R, Squires C, Mead GE, Religa D, Lundström E, Cheyne J, Wardlaw JM, Quinn TJ, Shenkin SD. Predicting post-stroke cognitive impairment using acute CT neuroimaging: a systematic review and meta-analysis. Int J Stroke. 2022;17(6):618–27. https://doi.org/10.1177/17474930211045836.

6 Brain Injury and Implications for Brain Health

Amy Y. Hao and Blessen C. Eapen

Key Points

1. Older adults are at high risk of experiencing TBI, resulting in death or disability.
2. A thorough evaluation is needed after traumatic injuries as symptoms may be delayed, obscured by medical comorbidities, or inaccurately attributed to normal aging.
3. Fall prevention is key to limiting the incidence of TBI in this population.

6.1 Introduction

Traumatic brain injury (TBI), known as the "silent epidemic," is a major cause of mortality and disability globally and is often unrecognized, unreported, and underdiagnosed. TBI is defined as a traumatically induced structural injury and/or physiological disruption of brain function as a result of an external force with a new onset of at least one of the following clinical signs immediately following the event: any period of loss of or a decreased level of consciousness; any loss of memory for events immediately before or after the injury; any alteration in mental state at the time of the injury; neurological deficits that may or may not be transient; intracranial lesion. TBI is categorized as mild, moderate, or severe based on the Glasgow Coma Scale (GCS) score, duration of loss of consciousness (LOC), post-traumatic amnesia (PTA), and alteration of consciousness (AOC) (Table 6.1) [1].

A. Y. Hao · B. C. Eapen (✉)
Polytrauma Network Site, Physical Medicine and Rehabilitation Service, VA Greater Los Angeles Healthcare System, Los Angeles, CA, USA

Department of Medicine, Division of Physical Medicine and Rehabilitation, David Geffen School of Medicine, University of California Los Angeles, Los Angeles, CA, USA
e-mail: amy.hao@va.gov; Blessen.Eapen2@va.gov

E. L. Cobbs, C. P. Prather (eds.), *Diseases of the Mind*, Topics in Geriatric Care,
https://doi.org/10.1007/978-981-97-5995-8_6

Table 6.1 Classification of TBI severity (If a patient meets criteria in more than one category of severity, the higher severity level is assigned)

Criteria	Mild	Moderate	Severe
Structural imaging	Normal	Normal or abnormal	Normal or abnormal
Loss of Consciousness (LOC)	0–30 min	>30 min and <24 hours	>24 hours
Alteration of consciousness/ mental state (AOC)[a]	up to 24 hours	>24 hours; severity based on other criteria	
Posttraumatic amnesia (PTA)	0–1 day	>1 and <7 days	>7 days
Glasgow Coma Scale (GCS) (best available score in first 24 hours)[b]	13–15	9–12	<9

[a]Alteration of mental status must be immediately related to the trauma to the head. Typical symptoms would be: looking and feeling dazed and uncertain of what is happening, confusion, difficulty thinking clearly or responding appropriately to mental status questions, and being unable to describe events immediately before or after the trauma event

[b]In April 2015, the DoD released a memorandum recommending against the use of GCS scores to diagnose TBI. See the memorandum for additional information [1]

An estimated 69 million people experience TBI worldwide each year. TBI is responsible for 30% of all injury-related deaths in the United States, and rates of death are highest in adults aged ≥75 years [2]. Road collisions are the most common cause of TBI in low- to middle-income countries [3]. In Europe, the most common mechanism of injury appears to be changing from traffic-related incidents to falls [4], particularly in high-income regions and among the older adult population [5].

Older adults may be at increased risk of TBI because of normal anatomical and physiological brain changes of aging, such as decreased brain volume/weight, vasculature, and cerebral autoregulation. Unintentional falls are the leading cause of TBI in older persons. Multiple factors increase the risk of falls, including medical comorbidities, age-related sensory impairments, polypharmacy, cognitive impairment, and neurological disorders. Active older adults may suffer sports-related injuries. Rates of TBI from skiing accidents are highest among skiers 55–64 years old [6].

Between 2007 and 2013, TBI-related hospitalizations and deaths increased as a result of falls in people ≥75 years old. Rates of hospitalization increase with age—those who are 85 years or older have a hospitalization rate four times that of 65–75-year-olds [7]. TBI in older adults leads to longer recovery and poorer functional outcomes [8]. Those who seek emergency care are more likely to require advanced imaging (head CT or brain MRI) and are four times more likely to be admitted for care in the intensive care unit, step-down unit or for surgery [9]. Rehospitalization due to complications and higher morbidity following a TBI is common [10].

Older people are more likely to be on anticoagulant or antiplatelet medications, and injuries such as cerebral contusions can be exacerbated by these medications leading to hemorrhagic conversion. Because of cerebral volume loss, the subdural space widens, placing increased stress on the bridging veins, leading to a higher incidence of shear injury and subdural hematomas even with minimal trauma. Because of the enlarged space, subdural blood may accumulate slowly, and clinical signs may not be evident immediately.

Older TBI survivors may have other conditions that require ongoing treatment, including direct physical, cognitive, and behavioral changes, as well as associated disease processes such as seizure disorders, respiratory problems, infections, and gastrointestinal or genitourinary issues. Older age and more severe functional impairments are risk factors for mortality [11]. Longitudinal studies show that older age and greater duration of injury chronicity were associated with greater disability, especially in TBI survivors over 75 years of age. This highlights the importance of assessing needs and providing rehabilitation treatments in the chronic phase of TBI [12].

6.2 Cognitive Disorders

6.2.1 Delirium

Delirium is characterized by an acute disturbance in attention and awareness with an additional disturbance in cognition [13]. In the United States, over 2.6 million adults over 65 years of age develop delirium each year [14]. It is present in one-third of hospitalized patients over 70 years old [15]. 75% of older patients with TBI in the intensive care unit develop delirium during their hospital stay. Up to 70% of patients transferred to inpatient neurorehabilitation for TBI suffer from delirium upon arrival. Duration of delirium is a predictor of worse long-term cognitive impairment [16].

Delirium is classified into hyperactive, hypoactive, and mixed delirium subtypes. Hypoactive delirium is particularly underrecognized and underdiagnosed and is associated with poorer prognosis [15]. Patients with acute neurologic injury who develop in-hospital delirium have an increased risk of long-term cognitive impairment [17].

6.2.2 Post-TBI Cognitive Impairments

It can be difficult to distinguish post-TBI cognitive impairments from premorbid mild cognitive impairment, as preinjury cognitive status is often unknown. Factors that can complicate cognitive assessment include other post-TBI sequelae, such as behavioral or mood disorders and sleep disturbance. Depressive disorders are common following TBI.

Older adults may need longer periods of rehabilitation to accommodate slower progress [18]. Factors that contribute to better cognitive gains include female sex, higher motor functioning at admission, longer length of stay, and care received at a freestanding rehabilitation facility [19].

Cognitive impairment post-TBI has also been associated with worse health-related quality of life [20]. Cognitive rehabilitation can improve executive functioning and affect daily living activities in older adults [21].

6.2.3 Neurodegenerative Disorders

TBI is thought to be a risk factor for dementia and neurodegenerative diseases such as Alzheimer's disease. However, results of studies on the relationship between TBI and cognitive impairment or dementia are mixed. In TBI survivors, age-related cognitive impairments may occur earlier in life, possibly due to post-TBI inflammatory changes leading to long-term microglial priming, which can impact behavioral and cognitive changes [22]. A history of TBI may lead to an earlier age of onset of cognitive impairment [23] but does not appear to be associated with progression from mild cognitive impairment to Alzheimer's dementia [24].

Some studies have not shown a correlation between TBI and dementia [25] or the rate of cognitive change [26]. The link between mild TBI and dementia is also unclear. While recent studies have suggested that mild TBI increases the incidence of dementia in adults ≥65 years old, it has not been associated with dementia risk in younger age groups.

Chronic traumatic encephalopathy (CTE) is a neurodegenerative process associated with repetitive TBI. It is diagnosed pathologically postmortem and is characterized by the accumulation of abnormal hyperphosphorylated tau in neurons, astrocytes, and cell processes around small vessels in an irregular pattern at the depths of the cortical sulci. Symptoms include mood, behavioral, cognitive, and motor changes. Evaluation of CTE pathological findings is more difficult in older adults due to the higher prevalence of coexisting age-related tau pathologies such as aging-related tau astrogliopathy (ARTAG) and primary age-related tauopathy (PART) [27].

6.3 Sleep

Sleep-wake disturbances are commonly reported following TBI. These can be manifestations of clinical syndromes, including insomnia, obstructive sleep apnea (OSA), and hypersomnias. A meta-analysis found the prevalence of sleep problems after TBI to be 50%, with 25–29% having a diagnosed sleep disorder [28]. These sleep disturbances can worsen other TBI-related symptoms, including attention and memory [29].

Sleep problems have been linked to cognitive dysfunction, functional impairment, and mood disturbances [30]. In the acute period post-TBI in hospitalized patients, sleep disruption is linked to both cognitive deficits and activities of daily living (ADL) dysfunction [31].

Changes that occur with sleep with normal aging are impacted by medical comorbidities such as diabetes, OSA, nocturia, pain symptoms, and dementia, as well as environmental and lifestyle factors. Older adults tend to have more frequent nighttime awakenings, reduced sleep duration, early morning awakenings, and relatively less time spent in deep sleep. Age-related circadian rhythm changes include the earlier shifts of sleep and wake time and a reduction in the amplitude of melatonin, core body temperature, and cortisol secretion [32].

The increased prevalence of sleep disorders amongst older adults places them at higher risk for TBI. Older adults with TBI have a higher incidence of sleep problems such as OSA, insomnia, and daytime sleepiness, which is also associated with lower quality of life measures [33]. Sleep problems have also been implicated in the development of dementia [34]. It has been suggested that sleep disturbances cause systemic inflammation, leading to increased beta-amyloid burden, which can contribute to the development of Alzheimer's disease [35]. Treatment of sleep-wake disorders can improve cognitive and communication outcomes measures [36].

CBT-I is an empirically validated brief psychotherapy treatment for insomnia and can be offered in an individual or group setting. Two reviews of the efficacy of CBT-I in the TBI population demonstrated a significant improvement in self-reported sleep outcomes [37, 38] as well as comorbid symptoms such as anxiety, depression, and pain. However, patients with severe cognitive impairment because of their TBI may not be good candidates for CBT-I. Pharmacological treatments must be weighed against potential medication side effects that can worsen post-TBI symptoms such as cognitive impairment, fatigue, dizziness, disorientation, and lowering of seizure threshold [39]. Complementary alternative medicine treatments such as acupuncture [40] and light therapy [41] have demonstrated positive effects on sleep symptoms in small studies.

6.4 Prevention

The growing incidence of TBI related to falls in older adults highlights the need to focus on fall prevention. In the United States, the Centers for Disease Control and Prevention STEADI (Stopping Elderly Accidents, Deaths & Injuries) program provides resources for healthcare providers to reduce fall risk (Table 6.2) [42].

Table 6.2 STEADI algorithm for fall risk screening, assessment, and interventions among community dwelling adults 65 years and older

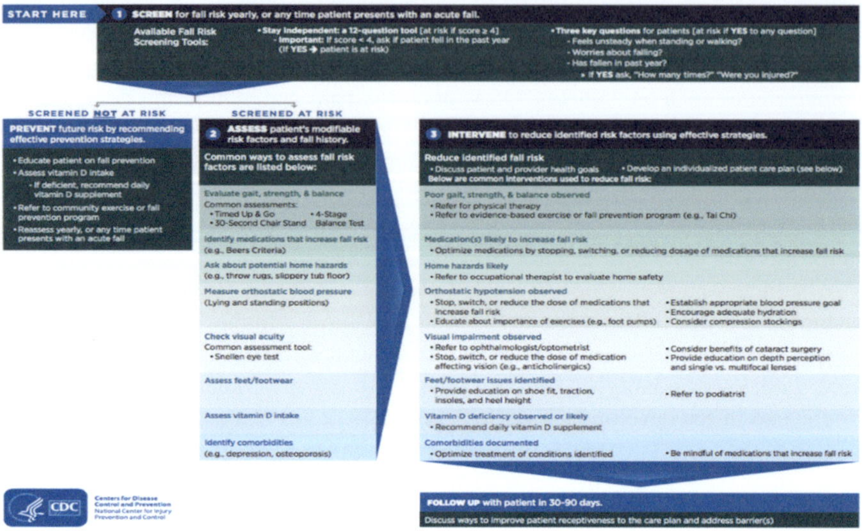

References

1. VA/DoD Clinical Practice Guideline for the Management and Rehabilitation of Post-acute Mild Traumatic Brain Injury. Healthquality.va.gov. https://www.healthquality.va.gov/guidelines/Rehab/mtbi/VADoDmTBICPGFinal508.pdf. Published 2022. Accessed 5 Aug 2022.
2. Surveillance Report of Traumatic Brain Injury-related Emergency Department Visits, Hospitalizations, and Deaths. Centers for Disease Control and Prevention, U.S. Department of Health and Human Services. 2014. https://www.cdc.gov/traumaticbraininjury/get_the_facts.html. Accessed 5 Aug 2022.
3. Dewan M, Rattani A, Gupta S, et al. Estimating the global incidence of traumatic brain injury. J Neurosurg. 2019;130(4):1080–97. https://doi.org/10.3171/2017.10.jns17352.
4. Brazinova A, Rehorcikova V, Taylor M, et al. Epidemiology of traumatic brain injury in Europe: a living systematic review. J Neurotrauma. 2021;38(10):1411–40. https://doi.org/10.1089/neu.2015.4126.
5. Peeters W, van den Brande R, Polinder S, et al. Epidemiology of traumatic brain injury in Europe. Acta Neurochir. 2015;157(10):1683–96. https://doi.org/10.1007/s00701-015-2512-7.
6. Xiang H, Kelleher K, Shields B, Brown K, Smith G. Skiing- and snowboarding-related injuries treated in U.S. emergency departments, 2002. J Trauma. 2005;58(1):112–8. https://doi.org/10.1097/01.ta.0000151270.26634.dd.
7. Taylor C, Bell J, Breiding M, Xu L. Traumatic brain injury–related emergency department visits, hospitalizations, and deaths—United States, 2007 and 2013. MMWR Surveillance Summaries. 2017;66(9):1–16. https://doi.org/10.15585/mmwr.ss6609a1.
8. LeBlanc J, Guise E, Gosselin N, Feyz M. Comparison of functional outcome following acute care in young, middle-aged and elderly patients with traumatic brain injury. Brain Inj. 2006;20(8):779–90. https://doi.org/10.1080/02699050600831835.
9. Pearson W, Sugerman D, McGuire L, Coronado V. Emergency department visits for traumatic brain injury in older adults in the United States: 2006–08. Western J Emerg Med. 2012;13(3):289–93. https://doi.org/10.5811/westjem.2012.3.11559.

10. Thompson H, Weir S, Rivara F, et al. Utilization and costs of health care after geriatric traumatic brain injury. J Neurotrauma. 2012;29(10):1864–71. https://doi.org/10.1089/neu.2011.2284.
11. Brooks J, Shavelle R, Strauss D, Hammond F, Harrison-Felix C. Life expectancy of 1-year survivors of traumatic brain injury, 1988–2019: updated results from the TBI model systems. Arch Phys Med Rehabil. 2022;103(1):176–9. https://doi.org/10.1016/j.apmr.2021.05.015.
12. Rabinowitz A, Kumar R, Sima A, et al. Aging with traumatic brain injury: deleterious effects of injury chronicity are most pronounced in later life. J Neurotrauma. 2021;38(19):2706–13. https://doi.org/10.1089/neu.2021.0038.
13. Petrucciani S, Recchia C. Diagnostic and statistical manual of mental disorders. 5th ed. American Psychiatric Association; 2013.
14. Oh E, Fong T, Hshieh T, Inouye S. Delirium in older persons. JAMA. 2017;318(12):1161. https://doi.org/10.1001/jama.2017.12067.
15. Marcantonio E. Delirium in hospitalized older adults. N Engl J Med. 2017;377(15):1456–66. https://doi.org/10.1056/nejmcp1605501.
16. Roberson S, Patel M, Dabrowski W, Ely E, Pakulski C, Kotfis K. Challenges of delirium management in patients with traumatic brain injury: from pathophysiology to clinical practice. Curr Neuropharmacol. 2021;19(9):1519–44. https://doi.org/10.2174/1570159x19666210119153839.
17. Meeks J, Bambhroliya A, Sheth S, et al. Long-term cognitive impairment associated with delirium in acute neurological injury. Crit Care Explor. 2020;2(6):e0130. https://doi.org/10.1097/cce.0000000000000130.
18. Hammond F, Baker-Sparr C, Dahdah M, et al. Predictors of 1-year global outcomes after traumatic brain injury among older adults: a NIDILRR traumatic brain injury model systems study. J Aging Health. 2019;31(10_suppl):68S–96S. https://doi.org/10.1177/0898264318819197.
19. Byom L, Zhao A, Yang Q, et al. Predictors of cognitive gains during inpatient rehabilitation for older adults with traumatic brain injury. PM R. 2023;15(3):265–77. https://doi.org/10.1002/pmrj.12795.
20. Gorgoraptis N, Zaw-Linn J, Feeney C, et al. Cognitive impairment and health-related quality of life following traumatic brain injury. NeuroRehabilitation. 2019;44(3):321–31. https://doi.org/10.3233/nre-182618.
21. Cisneros E, Beauséjour V, de Guise E, Belleville S, McKerral M. The impact of multimodal cognitive rehabilitation on executive functions in older adults with traumatic brain injury. Ann Phys Rehabil Med. 2021;64(5):101559. https://doi.org/10.1016/j.rehab.2021.101559.
22. Ziebell J, Rowe R, Muccigrosso M, et al. Aging with a traumatic brain injury: could behavioral morbidities and endocrine symptoms be influenced by microglial priming? Brain Behav Immun. 2017;59:1–7. https://doi.org/10.1016/j.bbi.2016.03.008.
23. Li W, Risacher S, McAllister T, Saykin A. Traumatic brain injury and age at onset of cognitive impairment in older adults. J Neurol. 2016;263(7):1280–5. https://doi.org/10.1007/s00415-016-8093-4.
24. LoBue C, Woon F, Rossetti H, Hynan L, Hart J, Cullum C. Traumatic brain injury history and progression from mild cognitive impairment to Alzheimer disease. Neuropsychology. 2018;32(4):401–9. https://doi.org/10.1037/neu0000431.
25. Grasset L, Glymour M, Yaffe K, et al. Association of traumatic brain injury with dementia and memory decline in older adults in the United States. Alzheimers Dementia. 2020;16(6):853–61. https://doi.org/10.1002/alz.12080.
26. Tripodis Y, Alosco M, Zirogiannis N, et al. The effect of traumatic brain injury history with loss of consciousness on rate of cognitive decline among older adults with normal cognition and Alzheimer's disease dementia. J Alzheimers Dis. 2017;59(1):251–63. https://doi.org/10.3233/jad-160585.
27. Bieniek K, Cairns N, Crary J, et al. The second NINDS/NIBIB consensus meeting to define neuropathological criteria for the diagnosis of chronic traumatic encephalopathy. J Neuropathol Exp Neurol. 2021; https://doi.org/10.1093/jnen/nlab001.

28. Mathias J, Alvaro P. Prevalence of sleep disturbances, disorders, and problems following traumatic brain injury: a meta-analysis. Sleep Med. 2012;13(7):898–905. https://doi.org/10.1016/j.sleep.2012.04.006.
29. Wilde M, Castriotta R, Lai J, Atanasov S, Masel B, Kuna S. Cognitive impairment in patients with traumatic brain injury and obstructive sleep apnea. Arch Phys Med Rehabil. 2007;88(10):1284–8. https://doi.org/10.1016/j.apmr.2007.07.012.
30. Albrecht J, Wickwire E. Sleep disturbances among older adults following traumatic brain injury. Int Rev Psychiatry. 2019;32(1):31–8. https://doi.org/10.1080/09540261.2019.1656176.
31. Duclos C, Beauregard M, Bottari C, Ouellet M, Gosselin N. The impact of poor sleep on cognition and activities of daily living after traumatic brain injury: a review. Aust Occup Ther J. 2014;62(1):2–12. https://doi.org/10.1111/1440-1630.12164.
32. Li J, Vitiello M, Gooneratne N. Sleep in normal aging. Sleep Med Clin. 2018;13(1):1–11. https://doi.org/10.1016/j.jsmc.2017.09.001.
33. Wei L, Wen Y, Thompson H, et al. Sleep disturbances following traumatic brain injury in older adults: a comparison study. J Head Trauma Rehabil. 2020;35(4):288–95. https://doi.org/10.1097/htr.0000000000000563.
34. Shi L, Chen S, Ma M, et al. Sleep disturbances increase the risk of dementia: a systematic review and meta-analysis. Sleep Med Rev. 2018;40:4–16. https://doi.org/10.1016/j.smrv.2017.06.010.
35. Irwin M, Vitiello M. Implications of sleep disturbance and inflammation for Alzheimer's disease dementia. Lancet Neurol. 2019;18(3):296–306. https://doi.org/10.1016/s1474-4422(18)30450-2.
36. Wiseman-Hakes C, Murray B, Moineddin R, et al. Evaluating the impact of treatment for sleep/wake disorders on recovery of cognition and communication in adults with chronic TBI. Brain Inj. 2013;27(12):1364–76. https://doi.org/10.3109/02699052.2013.823663.
37. Li X, Feng Y, Xia J, et al. Effects of cognitive behavioral therapy on pain and sleep in adults with traumatic brain injury: a systematic review and meta-analysis. Neural Plast. 2021;2021:1–12. https://doi.org/10.1155/2021/6552246.
38. Ludwig R, Vaduvathiriyan P, Siengsukon C. Does cognitive-behavioural therapy improve sleep outcomes in individuals with traumatic brain injury: a scoping review. Brain Inj. 2020;34(12):1569–78. https://doi.org/10.1080/02699052.2020.1831070.
39. Ouellet M, Beaulieu-Bonneau S, Morin C. Sleep-wake disturbances after traumatic brain injury. Lancet Neurol. 2015;14(7):746–57. https://doi.org/10.1016/s1474-4422(15)00068-x.
40. Zollman F, Larson E, Wasek-Throm L, Cyborski C, Bode R. Acupuncture for treatment of insomnia in patients with traumatic brain injury. J Head Trauma Rehabil. 2012;27(2):135–42. https://doi.org/10.1097/htr.0b013e3182051397.
41. Connolly L, Rajaratnam S, Murray J, Spitz G, Lockley S, Ponsford J. Home-based light therapy for fatigue following acquired brain injury: a pilot randomized controlled trial. BMC Neurol. 2021;21(1):262. https://doi.org/10.1186/s12883-021-02292-8.
42. Resource algorithm for fall risk screening, assessment, and intervention. STEADI—Older Adult Fall Prevention. https://www.cdc.gov/steadi/pdf/STEADI-Algorithm-508.pdf. Accessed 17 Sept 2022.

Mild Cognitive Impairment

7

Tania Alchalabi and Tahira I. Lodhi

Key Points

1. Mild cognitive impairment refers to the continuum of cognitive decline that is worse than baseline for an individual in one or more of the six cognitive domains; however, it does not amount to dementia.
2. Managing vascular risk factors by treating hypertension and diabetes and quitting smoking might reduce the chances of developing dementia.
3. Physicians can coach patients and families in prognostication related to MCI.

Mild cognitive impairment (MCI) refers to cognitive changes that are not typical of brain aging but do not meet the criteria of dementia [1]. Dementia onset happens when the instrumental activities of daily living become affected.

DSM-5 categorizes MCI as a mild neurocognitive disorder. It requires a subjective and objective decline from a baseline level of functioning in one or more of the six cognitive domains, namely learning and memory, social functioning, language, visuospatial function, complex attention, or executive functioning. It does not substantially interfere with instrumental activities of daily living and does not occur in the context of delirium or other psychological disorders [2].

T. Alchalabi (✉)
Memory Disorders Clinic, George Washington University, Washington, DC, USA
e-mail: talchalabi@mfa.gwu.edu

T. I. Lodhi
George Washington University, Washington, DC, USA
e-mail: tlodhi@mfa.gwu.edu

E. L. Cobbs, C. P. Prather (eds.), *Diseases of the Mind*, Topics in Geriatric Care,
https://doi.org/10.1007/978-981-97-5995-8_7

7.1 Amnestic Versus Non-amnestic

Amnestic MCI refers to impairment in one's ability to recall stored information, whereas non-amnestic MCI refers to impairment in one or more of the other cognitive domains while memory remains relatively intact. Non-amnestic cognitive decline is comparatively less common and often more difficult to diagnose than the amnestic form of MCI.

7.2 Epidemiology

The American Academy of Neurology updated its guidelines based on systematic reviews [3]. A lower education level was significantly associated with a higher prevalence of MCI. Two studies showed that male sex was associated with the presence of MCI, but other studies found similar baseline prevalence in men and women (Table 7.1).

7.3 Clinical Presentations

Patients may present with varied complaints depending on the cognitive domain affected. The levels of decline may not be comparable among different people because of the difference in baseline functional status. One or more cognitive domains may be affected. Learning new information is a particular challenge. A poignant example may be a 65-year-old data analyst who cannot memorize passwords or is having trouble learning new software. Patients may describe their condition as forgetting names or walking into a room and not knowing why they were there.

Case 1 An 80-year-old male, a retired college professor with a past medical history significant for hyperlipidemia, hypertension, and prediabetes, was seen in the memory clinic. He noted changes in remembering details of activities throughout the day. He was still capable of managing instrumental activities of daily living but needed more time to go through daily routines and had to write things down. Especially concerning was his inability to remember that medications that he had been taking for years. His partner had noticed memory changes for the last 2 years.

Table 7.1 Prevalence of mild cognitive impairment in older adults by age

Age (years)	Prevalence (%)
60–64	6.7
65–69	8.4
70–74	10.1
75–79	14.8
80–84	25.2

Note*:* MCI is common in older populations, and its prevalence increases with age

He drank a glass of wine with dinner and had a healthy diet. He quit smoking about 20 years ago. Before that he smoked a pack per day for 30 years. He did not exercise regularly.

His vital signs and physical examination were within normal limits. His laboratory evaluations, including a complete metabolic profile, complete biochemistry profile, thyroid function tests, and vitamin B12 levels, were all within normal limits. There was no evidence for Human Immunodeficiency Virus (HIV) or any other venereal disease. On cognitive assessment his score on the Montreal Cognitive Assessment was 28/30. Magnetic resonance imaging of his head showed microvascular ischemic changes throughout his brain.

Discussion This patient asked his geriatrician for a "memory pill." Although the US Food and Drug Administration has not approved any medication for MCI, it is important to listen to patients' concerns about cognitive changes and not mistakenly label them all as "normal aging." Besides obtaining a full evaluation through history and physical examination, getting a complete baseline laboratory evaluation to rule out reversible causes of cognitive impairment is imperative. Additionally, inquiring about and efficiently looking for risk factors for the development of cognitive impairment is important. The risk of small vessel disease increases steadily with age and is associated with a variety of systemic disorders, metabolic derangements, and lifestyle variables, including hypertension, chronic kidney disease, diabetes, alcohol use, and homocysteine levels [4].

Chronic hypertension leads to changes in cerebral blood flow autoregulation [5]. A shifted "set point" adapted to higher perfusion pressures also leads to an increased risk of symptomatic hypotension. Cautious use of antihypertensives is recommended as even short periodic hypotensive episodes contribute to white matter hyperintensities.

Physical activity may reduce the risk of dementia by increasing oxygen saturation and neurogenesis, decreasing vascular risk factors and inflammation [6]. Increased physical activity has been found to be associated with decreased progression of cognitive impairment to Alzheimer's Dementia [7]. Cardiovascular exercise is one of the few interventions that increases neuronal plasticity and replication, plays a role in neuroprotection, and has neuromodulation effects on chronic conditions. However, there is a lack of conclusive evidence, and more randomized controlled trials are needed [8]. Several meta-analyses and other published studies have shown the benefit of combined physical therapy and cognitive therapy. The primary analysis showed a small-to-medium positive effect of combined cognitive–physical interventions on global cognitive function in older adults with MCI [9].

Observational studies using dietary questionnaires to assess and quantify adherence to the Mediterranean diet in different population cohorts have found that patients who were most adherent to the diet had a lower incidence of mild cognitive impairment and AD and slower rates of cognitive decline compared with those who did not follow this diet [10]. It is worth mentioning the Keto Diet which is largely experimental currently. Ketone bodies, products of fat metabolism, are a source of energy for the brain and are available even when glucose supplies are insufficient (e.g., during severe carbohydrate restriction) or when its metabolism is defective, as in Alzheimer's Disease. This diet has been proposed as neuroprotective. In the last few years, some investigations have suggested that the ketogenic diet, which is characterized by high consumption of fat, moderate consumption of protein, and very low carbohydrate composition, may be useful for the prevention of age-associated cognitive decline. However, most available studies are experimental. Available data from clinical trials is not enough to draw definitive conclusions on the prevention and treatment of cognitive decline and Alzheimer's Disease [11].

The role coexistent of COPD and obstructive sleep apnea, referred to as overlap syndrome, in the development of mild cognitive impairment has been noted in the literature extensively. The more time spent at night with oxygen desaturation below 90% is associated with a higher incidence of MCI [12]. It is prudent for physicians to actively screen for sleep apnea while working up patients for possible etiologies for MCI.

This patient requested a "memory pill" from his geriatrician. Despite the US Food and Drug Administration not approving any medication for MCI, it's crucial to heed patients' concerns regarding cognitive changes and avoid mislabeling them as "normal aging." Apart from conducting a comprehensive evaluation involving history-taking, physical examination, and baseline laboratory tests to rule out reversible causes of cognitive impairment, it's essential to inquire about and efficiently assess risk factors for cognitive decline.

The risk of small vessel disease rises with age and is linked to various systemic disorders, metabolic imbalances, and lifestyle factors like hypertension, chronic kidney disease, diabetes, alcohol consumption, and homocysteine levels [4].

Chronic hypertension alters cerebral blood flow autoregulation [5], leading to a shifted "set point" adapted to higher perfusion pressures, thereby increasing the risk of symptomatic hypotension. It's advisable to cautiously use antihypertensives as periodic hypotensive episodes can contribute to white matter hyperintensities.

Physical activity may mitigate dementia risk by enhancing oxygen saturation and neurogenesis and reducing vascular risk factors and inflammation [6].

Increased physical activity correlates with a reduced progression of cognitive impairment to Alzheimer's Dementia [7].

Cardiovascular exercise boosts neuronal plasticity and replication, playing a role in neuroprotection and chronic condition management. However, conclusive evidence is lacking, necessitating more randomized controlled trials [8].

Combined physical and cognitive therapy interventions have shown a positive effect on global cognitive function in older adults with MCI [9].

Observational studies reveal that adherence to the Mediterranean diet is associated with a lower incidence of mild cognitive impairment and Alzheimer's disease, along with slower rates of cognitive decline [10].

The Keto Diet, though largely experimental, has been proposed as neuroprotective due to ketone bodies' role as an alternative brain energy source. Some studies suggest its potential for preventing age-associated cognitive decline, but conclusive evidence is lacking [11].

The coexistence of COPD and obstructive sleep apnea, known as overlap syndrome, is extensively noted in the literature for its association with mild cognitive impairment. Increased nocturnal oxygen desaturation correlates with a higher incidence of MCI, emphasizing the importance of screening for sleep apnea in patients being evaluated for cognitive impairment etiologies [12].Case 2 A 90-year-old female came to see a geriatrician for concerns about her memory. Her past medical history was significant for hypothyroidism, hypertension, depression, and anxiety. Her psychiatric conditions were not in full remission. She lived by herself in a retirement community. Prior to the Covid outbreak, she played tennis twice a week and was swimming three times a week. She also met regularly with her son and daughter who lived locally. When they were allowed to visit her in the facility, they noticed a significant decline in her memory. She was unable to remember her medications without writing down when she took them. Her vital signs, physical examination, and baseline laboratory workup were within normal limits. Her brain imaging did not show signs of cerebrovascular ischemia or hippocampal atrophy that might be related to Alzheimer's disease. Neuropsychological testing revealed uncontrolled anxiety and depression.

Discussion Major depressive disorder (MDD) is one of the most common psychiatric disorders worldwide [13]. In a systemic review done in 2018, the overall pooled prevalence of depression in patients with MCI was 32% [14]. In the USA, the lifetime prevalence of MDD exceeds 20% [15]. The World Health Organization ranks MDD as the leading cause of the global burden of disease. With ageing, factors such as social isolation, loneliness, and chronic medical problems might increase the overall impact of MDD [16].

Case 3 A 75-year-old male came in with his family after being diagnosed with mild cognitive impairment 2 years ago. He continued to be independent in instrumental activities of daily living; however, over the past 6–8 months, he found them more challenging. He took longer to finish a task at hand; even when he did that, he did not "trust" himself. At times, he asked his daughter to "double check." They scheduled this appointment with the patient's geriatrician to discuss prognosis, next steps, and goals of care.

Discussion Patients with MCI due to Alzheimer's Disease are more likely to progress to dementia than those with MCI that is not associated with toxic species of amyloid beta and/or the development of neurofibrillary tangles of hyperphosphorylated tau protein [17].

When counseling patients aged 65 years and older who are diagnosed with MCI that is suspected to be of neurodegenerative origin, the estimated risk of progression to dementia was found to be 10% per year. In one study, a community-based cohort of nondemented elderly people was followed longitudinally for 5 years. MCI was defined as memory complaints with objective memory impairment, without dementia, impairment of general cognitive functioning, or disability in activities of daily living. At baseline, there were 58 prevalent cases of MCI (2.8% of the sample). During a 5-year follow-up, 40 incident cases of MCI occurred in 1265 subjects at risk. The global incidence rate of MCI was 9.9/1000 person-years. MCI was a good predictor of Alzheimer's Disease with an annual conversion rate of 8.3% and a good specificity, but it was very unstable over time: Within 2–3 years, only 6% of the subjects continued to have MCI, whereas >40% reverted to normal [18].

The literature has reported an association between white matter lesions (WML) and mild cognitive impairment in T2-weighted images. Severe WML significantly increases the risk of mild cognitive impairment and dementia. This risk was higher in persons with low educational levels over a 7-year period. The people with a higher educational level had a higher cognitive reserve to be resilient against the deleterious effects of severe WML [19].

References

1. Sanford AM. Mild cognitive impairment. Clin Geriatr Med. 2017;33(3):325–37. https://doi.org/10.1016/j.cger.2017.02.005.
2. American Psychiatric Association. The diagnostic and statistical manual of mental disorders. 5th ed. American Psychiatric Association; 2013.
3. Petersen RC, Lopez O, Armstrong MJ, Getchius T, Ganguli M, Gloss D, Gronseth GS, Marson D, Pringsheim T, Day GS, Sager M, Stevens J, Rae-Grant A. Practice guideline update summary: Mild cognitive impairment: Report of the Guideline Development, Dissemination, and Implementation Subcommittee of the American Academy of Neurology. Neurology. 2018;90(3):126–35. https://doi.org/10.1212/WNL.0000000000004826.
4. Khan U, Porteous L, Hassan A, Markus HS. Risk factor profile of cerebral small vessel disease and its subtypes. J Neurol Neurosurg Psychiatry. 2007;78(7):702–6. https://doi.org/10.1136/jnnp.2006.103549.
5. Bowler JV. The concept of vascular cognitive impairment. J Neurol Sci. 2002;203-204:11–5. https://doi.org/10.1016/s0022-510x(02)00253-8.
6. Schmidt W, Endres M, Dimeo F, Jungehulsing GJ. Train the vessel, gain the brain: physical activity and vessel function and the impact on stroke prevention and outcome in cerebrovascular disease. Cerebrovasc Dis. 2013;35(4):303–12. https://doi.org/10.1159/000347061.
7. Scarmeas N, Luchsinger JA, Schupf N, Brickman AM, Cosentino S, Tang MX, Stern Y. Physical activity, diet, and risk of Alzheimer disease. JAMA. 2009;302(6):627–37. https://doi.org/10.1001/jama.2009.1144.

8. Demurtas J, Schoene D, Torbahn G, Marengoni A, Grande G, Zou L, Petrovic M, Maggi S, Cesari M, Lamb S, Soysal P, Kemmler W, Sieber C, Mueller C, Shenkin SD, Schwingshackl L, Smith L, Veronese N, European Society of Geriatric Medicine Special Interest Group in Systematic Reviews and Meta-Analyses, Frailty, Sarcopenia, and Dementia. Physical activity and exercise in mild cognitive impairment and dementia: an umbrella review of intervention and observational studies. J Am Med Dir Assoc. 2020;21(10):1415–1422.e6. https://doi.org/10.1016/j.jamda.2020.08.031.
9. Karssemeijer E, Aaronson JA, Bossers WJ, Smits T, Olde Rikkert M, Kessels R. Positive effects of combined cognitive and physical exercise training on cognitive function in older adults with mild cognitive impairment or dementia: a meta-analysis. Ageing Res Rev. 2017;40:75–83. https://doi.org/10.1016/j.arr.2017.09.003.
10. Estruch R, Ros E, Salas-Salvadó J, Covas MI, Corella D, Arós F, Gómez-Gracia E, Ruiz-Gutiérrez V, Fiol M, Lapetra J, Lamuela-Raventos RM, Serra-Majem L, Pintó X, Basora J, Muñoz MA, Sorlí JV, Martínez JA, Fitó M, Gea A, Hernán MA, et al. Primary prevention of cardiovascular disease with a Mediterranean diet supplemented with extra-virgin olive oil or nuts. N Engl J Med. 2018;378(25):e34. https://doi.org/10.1056/NEJMoa1800389.
11. Augustin K, Khabbush A, Williams S, Eaton S, Orford M, Cross JH, Heales S, Walker MC, Williams R. Mechanisms of action for the medium-chain triglyceride ketogenic diet in neurological and metabolic disorders. Lancet Neurol. 2018;17(1):84–93. https://doi.org/10.1016/S1474-4422(17)30408-8.
12. Wang Y, Li B, Li P, Gong T, Wu M, Fu J, Nie M, Dong Y, Hu K. Severe obstructive sleep apnea in patients with chronic obstructive pulmonary disease is associated with an increased prevalence of mild cognitive impairment. Sleep Med. 2020;75:522–30.
13. Kessler RC, Bromet EJ. The epidemiology of depression across cultures. Annu Rev Public Health. 2013;34:119–38. https://doi.org/10.1146/annurev-publhealth-031912-114409.
14. Ismail Z, Elbayoumi H, Fischer CE, Hogan DB, Millikin CP, Schweizer T, Mortby ME, Smith EE, Patten SB, Fiest KM. Prevalence of depression in patients with mild cognitive impairment: a systematic review and meta-analysis. JAMA Psychiatry. 2017;74(1):58–67. https://doi.org/10.1001/jamapsychiatry.2016.3162.
15. Hasin DS, Sarvet AL, Meyers JL, Saha TD, Ruan WJ, Stohl M, Grant BF. Epidemiology of adult DSM-5 major depressive disorder and its specifiers in the United States. JAMA Psychiatry. 2018;75(4):336–46. https://doi.org/10.1001/jamapsychiatry.2017.4602.
16. Hayley S, Hakim AM, Albert PR. Depression, dementia and immune dysregulation. Brain J Neurol. 2021;144(3):746–60. https://doi.org/10.1093/brain/awaa405.
17. Tahami Monfared AA, Byrnes MJ, White LA, Zhang Q. Alzheimer's disease: epidemiology and clinical progression. Neurol Ther. 2022;11(2):553–69. https://doi.org/10.1007/s40120-022-00338-8.
18. Larrieu S, Letenneur L, Orgogozo JM, Fabrigoule C, Amieva H, Le Carret N, Barberger-Gateau P, Dartigues JF. Incidence and outcome of mild cognitive impairment in a population-based prospective cohort. Neurology. 2002;59(10):1594–9. https://doi.org/10.1212/01.wnl.0000034176.07159.f8.
19. Mortamais M, Portet F, Brickman A, Provenzano F, Muraskin J, Akbaraly T, Berr C, Touchon J, Bonafe A, Bars E, Chamofluer N, Maller J, Meslin C, Sabatier R, Ritchie K, Artero S. Education modulates the impact of white matter lesions on the risk of mild cognitive impairment and dementia. Am J Geriatr Psychiatry. 2014;22(11):1336–45. https://doi.org/10.1016/j.jagp.2013.06.002.

Dementia Syndromes

8

Elizabeth Clark, Rachael Kantor, and Sophie Lin

Key Points

1. Dementia is a group of disorders characterized by the progressive decline in cognitive function that significantly impedes activities of daily living (ADLs).
2. Effective pharmacotherapy is extremely limited.
3. Nonpharmacologic modalities with proven efficacy in symptoms and behavior management include exercise, computerized cognitive training, massage/music therapy, and structured training for caregivers, but patients and caregivers often lack access to these.

8.1 Case 1

Ms. Johnson is a 72-year-old retired teacher. Widowed and childless, she remains close to her family and enjoys catching up with them at the annual family reunion.

This year, a construction detour confused her so much that she turned around and came home. The next day, her niece Jane found her aunt crying, and the apartment was awash in post-it notes: "Lock the door." "Put out the trash." "Pay the rent." Unpaid bills were neatly stacked beside the checkbook and utility cancellation notices.

The original version of the chapter has been revised. A correction to this chapter can be found at https://doi.org/10.1007/978-981-97-5995-8_12

E. Clark (✉)
Albert Einstein College of Medicine, Montefiore Medical Center, Bronx, NY, USA

R. Kantor
Department of Emergency Medicine, Kent Hospital, Warwick, RI, USA

S. Lin
New York Medical College, Metropolitan Hospital Center, New York, NY, USA

E. L. Cobbs, C. P. Prather (eds.), *Diseases of the Mind*, Topics in Geriatric Care,
https://doi.org/10.1007/978-981-97-5995-8_8

Recent events surprised her primary care physician of 30 years, "She's always been in good health, needs no medications. Never complained about memory problems."

Dementia workup supported Alzheimer's Dementia (AD) diagnosis:

Brain MRI: atrophy in the hippocampal and parietal areas.

Montreal Cognitive Assessment score: 15/30, notable deficits in memory and executive function.

Labs: normal, including B12, thyroid function tests (TFTs), HIV, and syphilis.

After caring for her mother with AD, Ms. Johnson prepared for the future. As Power-of-Attorney (POA) for finances and health care, Jane can manage Ms. Johnson's resources and honor her aunt's preferences for long-term care and her wishes for end-of-life (EOL) care.

8.2 Case 2

Mrs. Smith is a 69-year-old with hypertension, diabetes mellitus (DM), hyperlipidemia, hypothyroidism, and depression. A retired cook with a fifth-grade education, she has no toxic habits. She has an aunt with schizophrenia and a grandmother with depression.

She had followed regularly in psychiatry and primary care but stopped during the pandemic. She continued taking her antihypertensive and diabetes medications but discontinued her antidepressant.

Shortly after receiving her COVID-19 vaccine, Ms. Smith's depression and anxiety worsened. She confided in her son about children coming through the window at night, running around, and threatening her. There were no auditory hallucinations or suicidal ideation. She feels fine in the morning but becomes confused as the day progresses. She cries frequently, lacks motivation, is unable to remember new things, and sometimes does not recognize her children.

Her concerned son had her evaluated by psychiatry to address these new symptoms. The supported diagnosis: mixed Lewy Body (LBD) and Vascular Dementia (VaD).

Adjusted Mini Mental Status Exam (MMSE) score: 14/24.

Neurologic exam: non-focal.

Labs: normal, including B12, syphilis, and TFTs.

Brain MRI: moderate small vessel disease; lacunar infarcts; marked anterior bifrontal, bitemporal, and bi-frontoparietal cortical atrophy; moderate cerebellar atrophy.

Ms. Smith receives donepezil. Antipsychotic medications are avoided. Her family is counseled on the importance of hypertension and DM control and on cognitive-behavioral approaches to distressing behaviors.

Ms. Smith retains the capacity for some medical and financial decision-making. She appoints her son as healthcare agent, and her daughter as an alternate. She gives both children POA for finances. They arrange for bill payment and home care. They discuss her wishes for EOL care and complete the appropriate paperwork.

8.3 Case 3

Mr. Jones is a well-respected 57-year-old loan officer. Over the last year, his staff started noticing mistakes in loan applications. More recently, Mr. Jones, who never cursed, started making lewd remarks. He exposed himself during a staff meeting and was taken to the emergency room.

Assessment during a brief admission supported a diagnosis of frontotemporal dementia (FTD).

Cognitive testing: preserved memory but deficits in reasoning and executive function.

Neurologic exam: normal.

Labs: normal.

Brain MRI: frontal lobe atrophy.

Mr. Jones never completed a healthcare proxy or POA for finances and lacks the capacity to do so now. Mrs. Jones must apply for guardianship of her husband.

8.4 Introduction

Dementia is a group of disorders characterized by the progressive decline in cognitive function that significantly impedes activities of daily living (ADLs), leading to frailty, dependence, loss of personhood, and ultimately, death.

Dementia is one of the most challenging conditions faced by the aging population. Worldwide, approximately 50 million people have dementia, and that number is expected to increase to 82 million by 2030 and 152 million by 2050 [1]. AD comprises 60–70% of cases, followed by VaD, LBD, and FTD. Mixed dementias are also common, especially in older age.

While age is the greatest risk factor for dementia, dementia is not an inevitable consequence of aging. Truly reversible dementias are rarer than previously believed [2], but there are potentially modifiable risk factors that can affect dementia incidence and progression. These include less education, hypertension, hearing impairment, smoking, obesity, depression, physical inactivity, DM, low social contact, excessive alcohol intake, traumatic brain injury, and air pollution [3, 4]. A recent study found older adults who had COVID-19 infection were 50–80% more likely to have a new diagnosis of AD within the next year, with the highest risk females and those $\geq$85 [5].

Dementia evaluation requires a stepwise approach that includes presenting symptoms, clinical courses, careful history, and appropriate testing. Figure 8.1 is an algorithm for the outpatient dementia workup [6].

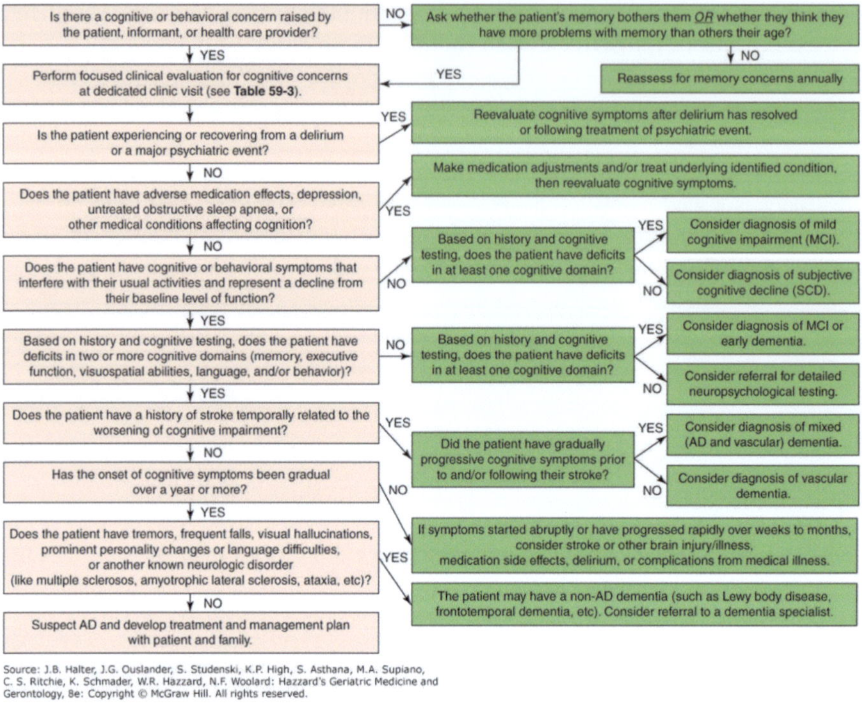

Fig. 8.1 Diagnostic algorithm for dementia (Used with permission)

8.5 Pathologies and Clinical Presentations

Dementia syndromes result from neurodegeneration through the deposition of abnormal proteins and/or vascular injury. While clinical features vary, there is considerable overlap among syndromes, and all can mimic psychiatric illnesses. Table 8.1 outlines the key characteristics of the major dementia syndromes. Familiarity with early signs of cognitive impairment can prompt timely workups that include attention to potentially modifiable conditions. Early detection affords patients, families, and providers a "window of opportunity" to plan for future care while patients retain the capacity to participate in decision-making and to complete legal documents. Accurate diagnosis helps prepare patients and families for what to expect as dementia syndrome unfolds and further allows providers to tailor treatments for the best long-term outcomes.

Table 8.1 Key features of major dementia syndromes

Syndrome	Alzheimer's disease [7–10]	Vascular dementia [11]	Dementia with lewy bodies [12–15]	Frontotemporal dementia [16–18]
				Behavioral variant (bv) Language variants (lv)
Epidemiology	Worldwide: 50 million cases	US/EU: 20% of dementias	10–15% of dementias	15–22/100,000 population
	US: 5.8 million European Union (EU): 9.1 million	Asia/developing countries: 30%		60% bvFTD, lvFTDs less common
Age	Prevalence(US):	Age distribution similar to stroke	Majority between 70 and 85	6th decade of life
	65–74: 5%			Rarely: Young-onset or older-onset
	75–84: 13%			
	≥85: 33%			
	Rare in younger people			
Risk factors	Age, family history, hearing loss, obesity, depression, head injury, low educational attainment, DM, hypertension, physical inactivity, down syndrome, apolipoprotein status, cerebral amyloidosis	Age, family hx hypertension, DM, hyperlipidemia, smoking, atrial fibrillation, congestive heart failure, stroke, hypo/hypercoagulability, connective tissue disorders, cancer, polycythemia	Genetics, age,rapid eye movement sleep behavior disorder (REM SBD)	Genetics

(continued)

Table 8.1 (continued)

Common presenting symptoms	Worsening of both the following over months to years:	Depends on brain area and neural pathways affected.	Dementia+:	bvFTD: Progressive deterioration of behavior and/or cognition:
	Amnesia: Impaired learning and recall of recently learned information	Deficits in attention, information processing, complex activity performance; disorganized thoughts; behavior problems; depression; apathy.	Fluctuations	Behavioral disinhibition
	Plus impairment in 1+ cognitive domains:	Less common: Hallucinations, delusions	Visual hallucinations	Apathy/inertia.
	Language (especially word-finding)	Stepwise deficit development	Parkinsonism	Loss of sympathy/empathy
	Visuospatial (especially spatial recognition)		REM SBD	Compulsive behavior
	Executive function (especially reasoning, judgment, problem-solving)		Attention, executive function, visual processing deficits	Hyperorality or dietary changes
				Dysexecutive syndrome
Disease progression	Memory loss	Progression rarely slowed with vascular risk factor control.	Spatial and perceptual difficulties occur early	bvFTD: Progressive deterioration in social function and personality
	Difficulty performing ADLs		Daytime sleepiness	Insidious decline in language skills (lv)
	Inability to plan/problem-solve		Complex visual hallucinations	Memory and visuospatial function spared until late disease
	Decreased/poor judgment		Parkinsonism	
	Mood/personality changes		Supportive features: Daytime somnolence, hyposmia, severe antipsychotic sensitivity	
	Weight loss/physical decline			
	Behavioral problems increasing caregiver burden			

(continued)

Imaging abnormalities	Amyloid on PET imaging	Lacunar, or macro/microinfarction	Low dopamine transporter uptake in basal ganglia PET and SPECT imaging	Hypometabolism on FDG-PET in the frontal brain
	Decreased fluorodeoxyglucose (FDG) uptake on PET in temporo–parietal cortex	White matter hyperintensities	Low uptake iodine^{123} MIBG myocardial scintigraphy	Frontal hypoperfusion on HMPAO-SPECT
	Disproportionate atrophy on structural magnetic resonance imaging in medial, basal, and lateral temporal lobe, and medial parietal cortex			
Neuropathology	Decades-long 42 amino-acid long amyloid- β (Aβ) protein accumulation in extracellular brain plaques.	Macroinfarction: Often middle cerebral artery distribution	Lewy bodies and neurites due to protein misfolding/alpha-synuclein accumulation → cellular injury/neuronal degeneration	Frontotemporal lobar degeneration,intranuclear inclusions: Tau, TDP-43 or occasionally fused in sarcoma (FUS).
	Hyperphosphorylation and tau secretion → intraneuronal neurofibrillary tangles.	Embolic strokes		
	Apoprotein E4, major genetic risk factor for early onset disease	Small-vessel disease: Microinfarction, microbleeds, lacunar infarcts		
		White matter degeneration		

8.6 Treatment Options and Limitations

Effective pharmacotherapy in dementia is extremely limited. Many commonly prescribed and over-the-counter medications (especially anticholinergics) and recreational substances increase dementia risk and worsen symptoms [19]. Table 8.2 outlines medications currently available.

Nonpharmacologic modalities with proven efficacy in symptoms and behavior management include exercise, computerized cognitive training, massage/music therapy, and structured training for caregivers. Despite their benefits, patients and caregivers often lack access to these interventions [20–22].

Table 8.2 Drugs used in dementia

Drug class	Use	Benefits	Side effects	Caution
Acetylcholinesterase inhibitors: Donepezil, Rivastigmine, Galantamine	Mild to moderate AD	MMSE score stable for a year vs. 2 to 3 point decline in placebo group	Gastrointestinal (cramps, nausea, diarrhea), vivid dreams, urinary incontinence, bradycardia/arrhythmia, syncope	May worsen FTD
	Also VaD and LBD	May help with behavior problems		
NMDA blockers: Memantine	Moderate to severe Alzheimer dementia	Small improvement in global clinical rating scales in moderate to severe AD	Dizziness, constipation, diarrhea, headache, somnolence	May worsen FTD
		No improvement in mild AD		
Aducanumab: Monoclonal antibody targeting amyloid beta	May only be used in MCI or mild dementia	Reduced Aβ plaques on PET scan but showed clinical improvement only with the higher dose in one of two trials	Must have MRI of brain at baseline and at intervals to monitor for amyloid-related imaging abnormalities (ARIA), which may include microhemorrhages and vasogenic edema	Biomarker confirmation of Aβ using CSF or PET must be made prior to initiating treatment
	First approved disease-modifying AD therapy			Given as monthly intravenous infusions
Antidepressants	Coexisting depression	May improve depressive symptoms and function	Vary with specific antidepressant	Depression treatment unlikely to reverse all cognitive impairment

(continued)

Table 8.2 (continued)

Drug class	Use	Benefits	Side effects	Caution
Antipsychotics	Last resort for behavioral issues	May improve distressing behaviors	Extrapyramidal side effects, sedation	Black box warning: Increased risk of death
			Can precipitate irreversible parkinsonian symptoms, especially in LBD	Avoid older agents (haloperidol)
				Dosing: Start low, go slow
Other medications or dietary supplements: 3-hydroxy-3-methylglutaryl reductase inhibitors, non-steroidal anti-inflammatory drugs, vitamins, dietary supplements, stop antihypertensive medications	Patient/family choice	No evidence-based improvements	Varies with specific treatment	Drug-drug and drug-disease interactions

8.7 Associated syndromes

Hearing Loss Hearing impairment has a complex relationship with dementia development. Central auditory degeneration worsens peripheral deafness, decreases compensatory hearing mechanisms, and impairs cognition. Central auditory dysfunction may be an early presentation of neurodegenerative dementias [23].

Delirium Delirium is an acute, fluctuating mental status change associated with inattention and alteration in cognition occurring over a short time. Any cognitive impairment increases the risk of delirium in the ICU and other acute settings. Even without a prior diagnosis of dementia, delirium is a predictor of future cognitive decline [24, 25]. Delirium superimposed on dementia has a high prevalence among hospitalized older patients, increasing length of stay, physical and cognitive decline, and risk of institutionalization [26].

Depression Depression is associated with mild cognitive impairment (MCI) and dementia, often preceding or coinciding with a dementia diagnosis. More research is needed to develop treatments for the intersection of these two conditions [27].

Disability and Death Dementia increases mortality and institutionalization among hip fracture patients [28]. Dementia worsens function and increases death rates from COVID-10 infections among older adults [29].

Nutrition Eating problems are common across dementia syndromes. Tube feeding has long been proffered as a solution despite evidence to the contrary. A recent Cochrane Review again reported no evidence that tube feeding improves nutritional status, decreases pain, or decreases mortality, but good evidence that it increases the risk of pressure ulcers [30].

8.8 Conclusion

All dementia syndromes rob people of their humanity, burden caregivers, and hasten death. Truly reversible forms of dementia are exceedingly rare; many factors are modifiable. Early detection allows patients, families, and providers to assess needs and make EOL plans while patients can participate in decision-making. Accurate diagnoses help map the specific road ahead and facilitate treatment decisions to minimize symptoms, prevent harm, and improve the quality of life for patients and their caregivers.

References

1. Risk reduction of cognitive decline and dementia: WHO guidelines. World Health Organization. https://www.who.int/publications-detail-redirect/9789241550543. Accessed 15 July 2022.
2. Clarfield AM. The decreasing prevalence of reversible dementias: an updated meta-analysis. Arch Intern Med. 2003;163(18):2219–29.
3. Livingston G, et al. Dementia prevention, intervention, and care: 2020 report of the lancet commission. Lancet. 2020;396:413–46.
4. Loscalzo J, et al. Harrison's principles of internal medicine. 21st ed. New York: McGraw-Hill; 2022.
5. Wang L, et al. Association of COVID-19 with new-onset Alzheimer's disease. J Alzheimers Dis. 2022;89:411–4.
6. Halter JB, et al. Dementia including Alzheimer's disease. In: Hazzard's geriatric medicine and gerontology. McGraw-Hill; 2022.
7. Zetterberg H, et al. Biomarkers for Alzheimer's disease-preparing for a new era of disease-modifying therapies. Mol Psychiatry. 2021;26(1):296–308.
8. McKhann GM, et al. The diagnosis of dementia due to Alzheimer's disease: recommendations from the National Institute on Aging-Alzheimer's Association workgroups on diagnostic guidelines for Alzheimer's disease. Alzheimers Dement. 2011;7(3):263–9.
9. Atri A. The Alzheimer's disease clinical Spectrum: diagnosis and management. Med Clin N Am. 2019;103:263–93.
10. Alzheimer's Association. 2022 Alzheimer's Disease facts and figures. https://www.alz.org/media/Documents/alzheimers-facts-and-figures.pdf.
11. Bir SC, et al. Emerging concepts in vascular dementia: a review. J Stroke Cerebrovasc Dis. 2021;30(8):105864.
12. Abe K. Reader response: diagnosis and management of dementia with Lewy bodies: fourth consensus report of the DLB consortium. Neurology. 2018;90(6):298–9.
13. Cummings JL. Dementia with lewy bodies: molecular pathogenesis and implications for classification. J Geriatr Psychiatry Neurol. 2004;17(3):112–9.
14. McKeith I, et al. Diagnosis and management of dementia with Lewy bodies: fourth consensus report of the DLB consortium. Neurology. 2017;89(1):88–100.
15. Prasad S, et al. Recent advances in Lewy body dementia: a comprehensive review. Dis Mon. 2023;69(5):101441. https://doi.org/10.1016/j.disamonth.2022.101441.
16. Piguet O, et al. Behavioural-variant frontotemporal dementia: an update. Dement Neuropsychol. 2013;7(1):10–8.

17. Rascovsky K, et al. Sensitivity of revised diagnostic criteria for the behavioural variant of frontotemporal dementia. Brain. 2011;134:2456–77.
18. Onyike CU, et al. The epidemiology of frontotemporal dementia. Int Rev Psychiatry. 2013;25(2):130–7. https://doi.org/10.3109/09540261.2013.776523.
19. Zheng YB, et al. Anticholinergic drugs and the risk of dementia: a systematic review and meta-analysis. Neurosci Biobehav Rev. 2021;127:296–306.
20. Ströhle A, et al. Drug and exercise treatment of Alzheimer disease and mild cognitive impairment: a systematic review and meta-analysis of effects on cognition in randomized controlled trials. Am J Geriatr Psychiatry. 2015;23:1234–49.
21. Liang JH, et al. Comparison of multiple interventions for older adults with Alzheimer disease or mild cognitive impairment: a PRISMA-compliant network meta-analysis. Medicine (Baltimore). 2018;97(20):e10744.
22. Watt JA, et al. Comparative efficacy of interventions for aggressive and agitated behaviors in dementia: a systematic review and network meta-analysis. Ann Intern Med. 2019;171:633–42.
23. Johnson JCS, et al. Hearing and dementia: from ears to brain. Brain. 2021;144(2):391–401.
24. Fong TG, et al. The interface between delirium and dementia in elderly adults. Lancet Neurol. 2015;14(8):823–32.
25. Mart MF, et al. ICU survivorship-the relationship of delirium, sedation, dementia, and acquired weakness. Crit Care Med. 2021;49(8):1227–40.
26. Han QYC, et al. Prevalence, risk factors, and impact of delirium in hospitalized older adults with dementia: a systematic review and meta-analysis. J Am Med Dir Assoc. 2022;23(1):23–32.e27.
27. Leyhe T, et al. A common challenge in older adults: classification, overlap, and therapy of depression and dementia. Alzheimers Dement. 2017;13(1):59–71.
28. Jorissen RN, et al. Effect of dementia on outcomes after surgically treated hip fracture in older adults. J Arthroplasty. 2021;36(9):3181–3186.e4.
29. Hariyanto TI, et al. Dementia and outcomes from coronavirus disease 2019 (COVID-19) pneumonia: a systematic review and meta-analysis. Arch Gerontol Geriatr. 2021;93:104299.
30. Davies N, et al. Enteral tube feeding for people with severe dementia. Cochrane Database Syst Rev. 2021;8(8):CD013503.

9 Living with Dementia and Cognitive Disorders: Beyond Pharmacology

Jiska Cohen-Mansfield

Key Points

- Behavioral challenges refer to inappropriate behaviors manifested by persons with dementia, which include physical nonaggressive behaviors, such as repetitive wandering; verbal behaviors, like repeated requests for help or attention; and aggressive behaviors, like screaming or hitting.
- Of multiple theoretical frameworks addressing the reasons for behavioral challenges, the "unmet needs" theory is best supported by research evidence.
- The most common unmet needs are relief of pain and/or discomfort, relief of boredom, and social engagement to reduce feelings of isolation and loneliness. There is a statistical relationship between the type of behavioral challenge and the most likely unmet need underlying it.
- Systemic transformation is needed in the resources provided for the care and the way in which care is delivered to minimize behavioral challenges. Greater emphasis on preventive care is required to address unmet needs before they manifest in behavioral challenges.

J. Cohen-Mansfield (✉)
Department of Health Promotion, School of Public Health, Sackler Faculty of Medicine, Tel Aviv University, Tel Aviv, Israel

Minerva Center for Interdisciplinary Study of End of Life, Tel Aviv University, Tel Aviv, Israel

Igor Orenstein Chair for the Study of Geriatrics, Tel Aviv University, Tel Aviv, Israel
e-mail: jiska@tauex.tau.ac.il

E. L. Cobbs, C. P. Prather (eds.), *Diseases of the Mind*, Topics in Geriatric Care,
https://doi.org/10.1007/978-981-97-5995-8_9

9.1 Introduction

A recent study [1], which involved interviews with an array of nursing home staff, from CEOs to nursing aids at five Israeli nursing homes, revealed a common complaint: residents' aggressive behavior. Routine practice in morning care involved nursing aids waking residents starting at 5:30 am in order to shower, dress, and seat them in the dining room by 8:00 am. The staff noted aggression by residents during early morning care, but they did not recognize the association between the residents' aggressiveness and the staff's morning care practices. This is, but one example of insufficiently informed care practices and systems that lead to the very problem that all agree needs to be remedied. This chapter (1) summarizes the behavioral challenges of persons with dementia, (2) describes the main conceptual and practical ways to address them without resorting to pharmacological means, and (3) discusses systemic and structural changes needed to improve care-recipients' and caregivers' well-being.

"Dementia" refers to a group of syndromes that involve a significant deterioration of memory and a decline in at least one other cognitive function, such as language or executive function [2]. In addition to memory problems, persons with dementia commonly experience difficulties with concentration and orientation, as well as a gradual decline in the ability to perform activities of daily living, starting with more complex tasks like money management and, later on, simpler tasks. Long-term memory is usually preserved much longer than short-term memory; procedural memory (how to do something) is preserved much longer than explicit (or declarative) memory (memory of factual information). Persons with dementia tend to retain their sense of identity longer than the people around them judge it to be retained [3].

9.2 Behavioral Challenges

The terms "agitation," "challenging behavior," and "problematic behavior" will be used interchangeably. Such behavior can be verbal or physical, aggressive or nonaggressive, and may be repetitive, like wandering around much of the time or repeatedly asking a question. The behavior can involve actions inappropriate to the circumstances, like urinating in a flower pot in a common area. Multiple studies examining the frequency of such behavior identified three main syndromes: aggressive behavior like hitting another person; physically nonaggressive behavior like repeatedly moving objects from place to place; and verbal/vocal behavior like repetitive complaining or screaming [4].

Neuropsychiatric symptoms in dementia [5] usually include the following 12 conditions: delusions, hallucinations, agitation/aggression, depression, anxiety, euphoria, apathy, disinhibition, irritability, aberrant motor behavior, sleep problems, and eating disorders. These conditions or characteristics, however, are not necessarily related to each other, with each being worthy of a study concerning whether it is more prevalent in dementia. As to conditions found to be prevalent, the next questions are: at what stages of dementia do they tend to occur, with what common etiologies, and what effective treatment can be provided? Other than agitation/aggression, these conditions are not behavior challenges and will not be addressed here.

9.3 Theoretical Frameworks and Their Implications for Prevention and Treatment

Several etiological theoretical models have been proposed for explaining behavioral challenges, including neurobiological changes, e.g. [6], with the implication that psychotropic medications are appropriate for prevention and treatment; a behavioral model which emphasizes triggers and consequences, e.g. [7], suggesting that a change in either antecedent to, or reactions to the behavior should be implemented as prevention or treatment; and a reduced stress threshold in dementia, e.g. [8]. pointing to a reduction of noise and other stimuli as a path to prevention and treatment.

Yet the theoretical model that best fits available research findings is that of the "unmet needs" model [9], which posits that persons with dementia experience unmet needs due to a combination of their decreased abilities, their environment's limitations in understanding their needs and addressing them, and a mismatch between their environment and the characteristics of their past and current life experience. Older persons with dementia often retain many habits and preferences, yet the dementia disease process limits their physical and cognitive abilities, both to communicate their needs and to address them. Challenging behavior may manifest in an effort to meet unmet needs, such as in the person who moves things from one place to another *to meet a need* for activity. Repeatedly asking for help may also be an effort *to communicate an unmet need.* Alternatively, challenging behavior may be a *direct outcome of an unmet need*, like crying due to untreated pain.

Fundamentally, the unmet needs model is based on the recognition that there is no difference between the needs of persons with dementia and those of the general population. All have needs for security, nutrition, love, and meaningful occupation. The difference between persons with dementia and others is that the former experience decreasing levels of ability to articulate and meet those needs, resulting in reliance upon people in their social environment to detect and address the needs. A prerequisite for addressing people's needs is understanding the nature of the most common ones: the need to alleviate pain and discomfort, to reduce loneliness and enhance social contact, including giving and receiving love and affection, and the need to reduce boredom through activity and stimulation [10].

9.4 Types of Unmet Needs and Implications for Prevention and Treatment

The unmet needs model informs directions for intervention and prevention and recognizes that each type of need may be addressed in multiple ways.

Pain and Discomfort Pain needs to be assessed both as to its level and its source. Pain evaluation usually relies heavily on persons having sufficient verbal communication skills to describe their pain. For those persons who cannot communicate sufficiently, specialized assessment tools have been developed and validated [11]. Treatment of pain can involve examination to find its location (overgrown nail, gum abscess, etc.), directly treating the source of pain, or using analgesic medication. Discomfort can involve a range of environmental and care issues, including awkward seating position, use of restraints, unresponsive care practices like ignoring requests for a drink or help getting to the bathroom [12], and other deficits in care [13].

Boredom Versus Engagement In addressing boredom or the need for engagement, the multiple approaches available include providing *active* stimulation like activity programs, e.g. exercise, dancing, singing, creative arts, etc., or walking. Such activities rely on long-term memory and procedural memory to enhance the level of engagement and enjoyment derived from the activity. Another approach is enabling *passive* stimulation. Many persons with dementia receive minimal stimulation because of unaddressed sensory problems like the inadequacy of or loss of eyeglasses or hearing aids. Ameliorating such sensory deficits will immediately render the available environmental stimulation accessible. Sensory interventions like music and massage can also be used. For those persons with dementia whose problematic behavior constitutes their way of addressing unmet needs, strategies that accommodate such behavior can be particularly helpful. Accommodating behaviors like pacing and wandering usually involves strategies to reduce risks, such as camouflaging doors from which persons with dementia might exit to a dangerous environment or decreasing the risk of falls by minimizing hazards like unsecured area rugs, stray wiring, and wet or slippery floors. Another accommodation is to change the environment to make it more acceptable, like escorting a person who tends to pace to a park or giving a person who tends to fidget with papers or a diaper more socially appropriate objects to handle.

Loneliness Versus Social Relationships The last group of unmet needs involves the need to have social contact and avoid loneliness. Here too, there is a range of options. The most potent is one-on-one social interaction about topics of interest to the individual. While effective, this is often unfeasible on a regular basis. Group activities present an effective and more realistic alternative [14], and their effects can be optimized by preparing materials that are more likely to engage the person with dementia and that are presented by activity group leaders who are enthusiastic and compassionate. Technological solutions can also be helpful, including simulated presence therapy [15], videotapes of family members talking to the person with dementia [16], and commercially available videos of talking to the person with dementia. Other approaches include pet therapy involving visits by dogs or cats [17], socially assistive pet robots [18], and the use of dolls, particularly those that look like real babies [19]. Anecdotally, other stimuli have been found to provide an enhanced sense of social contact, as in persons who befriend their image in the mirror. All interventions require a holistic ethical examination to ensure that the intervention is beneficial for the person with dementia and does not negatively affect relationships within an existing social network.

The response to different types of stimuli is affected by the person's characteristics, including level of cognitive function [20], personal preferences [21], and sense of identity [3]. The response is also affected by the environmental background, such as noise level [22], and by stimulus characteristics in that social stimuli are often more engaging than nonsocial ones [23].

9.5 Efficacy and Effectiveness

Most of these strategies have been studied using one or more intervention approaches at a time. There are, however, studies that aimed to examine the global approach, and those generally fit into two categories: (1) studies that examined each individual with dementia for causes of challenging behavior, the likely unmet needs, and potential strategies to address the behavior, e.g. [24], and (2) studies that took a more global approach, like teaching staff representatives how to use an unmet needs strategy, and how to train the rest of the staff in its use, e.g. [25]. Both approaches found significant reductions in challenging behavior and improvement in the quality of life of the persons with dementia who received the interventions. The first approach was conducted in a research rather than practice context, while the second approach required a sizeable investment in the mentoring of staff, e.g. [26], and achieved only limited sustainability due to staff turnover and other systemic difficulties, e.g. [1].

9.6 Future Directions

The most important challenge in this field is the translation of available research findings into everyday practice. Examples include instituting regular checks to detect pain and discomfort, care enhancement to address discomfort (whether due to illness or deficient care), improvement in practices to engage persons with dementia in meaningful activities and provision of regular supportive social contact. Prior efforts in these directions have resulted in meaningful progress yet have fallen short of what is truly needed. Systemic factors appear to pose barriers to further progress. Competing societal priorities and financial demands have resulted in insufficient resources and staffing for the care of persons with dementia. Healthcare policy tends to venerate a medical model of care rather than focusing on well-being, examining diagnoses rather than delving into people's unmet needs. The current paradigm may partially explain the absence of personnel with expertise in dementia care in most places responsible for such care.

A basic transformation is needed. In addition to the systemic issues enumerated above, a change of direction is needed in how transforming care is undertaken. Future efforts need to focus on developing an alternative type of care, one that will be conducive both to the care-recipient and caregiver. Rather than merely *instructing* staff/caregivers in the principles of good care, we need to *work with* staff and provide them with materials that reflect recent research, as well as systems that are oriented toward a higher level of care. For example, since most activity personnel possess neither the knowledge, time, nor resources to prepare optimal materials for activities for persons with dementia, funders and administrators should supply appropriate materials and institute measures to ensure correct use. Such improved strategies and systems result not only in improved care practices, reduction in agitated behaviors, and increased well-being for nursing home residents but also in making the work easier and more pleasurable for the staff or other caregivers, increasing their own well-being and job satisfaction.

References

1. Cohen-Mansfield J, Meschiany G. Israeli nursing home staff perspectives on challenges to quality care for residents with dementia. Geriatr Nurs. 2022;44:15–23.
2. APA Dictionary of Psychology. American Psychological Association. https://dictionary.apa.org/dementia. Accessed 2 Aug 2022.
3. Cohen-Mansfield J, Parpura-Gill A, Golander H. Salience of self-identity roles in persons with dementia: differences in perceptions among elderly persons, family members and caregivers. Soc Sci Med. 2006;62(3):745–57.
4. Rabinowitz J, Davidson M, De Deyn PP, Katz I, Brodaty H, Cohen-Mansfield J. Factor analysis of the Cohen-Mansfield Agitation Inventory in three large samples of nursing home patients with dementia and behavioral disturbance. Am J Geriatr Psychiatry. 2005;13(11):991–8.
5. Lyketsos CG, Lopez O, Jones B, Fitzpatrick AL, Breitner J, DeKosky S. Prevalence of neuropsychiatric symptoms in dementia and mild cognitive impairment results from the cardiovascular health study. JAMA. 2002;288(12):1475–83.
6. Craig D, Hart DJ, Carson R, McIlroy SP, Passmore AP. Allelic variation at the A218C tryptophan hydroxylase polymorphism influences agitation and aggression in Alzheimer's disease. Neurosci Lett. 2004;363(3):199–202.
7. Dobbs D, Zimmerman S, Carder P, Beeber AS, Palmertree SJ. Staff reports of behavioral expressions of persons with dementia in 250 assisted living communities. Gerontologist. 2022;62(2):169–80.
8. Hall GR, Buckwalter KC. Progressively lowered stress threshold: a conceptual model for care of adults with Alzheimer's disease. Arch Psychiatr Nurs. 1987;1(6):399–406.
9. Cohen-Mansfield J. Theoretical frameworks for behavioral problems in dementia. Alzheimers Care Today. 2000;1(4):8–21.

10. Cohen-Mansfield J, Dakheel-Ali M, Marx MS, Thein K, Regier NG. Which unmet needs contribute to behavior problems in persons with advanced dementia? Psychiatry Res. 2015;228(1):59–64.
11. Cohen-Mansfield J, Lipson S. The utility of pain assessment for analgesic use in persons with dementia. Pain. 2008;134(1–2):16–23.
12. Cohen-Mansfield J, Thein K, Marx MS, Dakheel-Ali M, Jensen B. Sources of discomfort in persons with dementia: scale and initial results. Behav Neurol. 2015;2015:732832.
13. Cohen-Mansfield J, Parpura-Gill A. Bathing: a framework for intervention focusing on psychosocial, architectural and human factors considerations. Arch Gerontol Geriatr. 2007;45(2):121–35.
14. Cohen-Mansfield J. The impact of group activities and their content on persons with dementia attending them. Alzheimers Res Ther. 2018;10(1):37.
15. Abraha I, Rimland JM, Lozano-Montoya I, et al. Simulated presence therapy for dementia. Cochrane Database Syst Rev. 2020;4(4):CD011882.
16. Werner P, Cohen-Mansfield J, Fischer J, Segal G. Characterization of family-generated videotapes for the management of verbally disruptive behaviors. J Appl Gerontol. 2000;19(1):42–57.
17. Marx MS, Cohen-Mansfield J, Regier NG, Dakheel-Ali M, Srihari A, Thein K. The impact of different dog-related stimuli on engagement of persons with dementia. Am J Alzheimers Dis Other Dement. 2010;25(1):37–45.
18. Bradwell H, Edwards KJ, Winnington R, Thill S, Allgar V, Jones RB. Exploring the effect of implementing affordable socially assistive pet robots in eight care homes before and during the COVID-19 pandemic: a stratified cluster randomised controlled trial and mixed-method study. JMIR Aging. 2022;5(3):e38864.
19. Martín-García A, Corregidor-Sánchez AI, Fernández-Moreno V, Alcántara-Porcuna V, Criado-Álvarez JJ. Effect of doll therapy in behavioral and psychological symptoms of dementia: a systematic review. Healthcare (Basel). 2022;10(3):421.
20. Cohen-Mansfield J, Marx MS, Regier NG, Dakheel-Ali M. The impact of personal characteristics on engagement in nursing home residents with dementia. Int J Geriatr Psychiatry. 2009;24(7):755–63.
21. Cohen-Mansfield J, Marx MS, Thein K, Dakheel-Ali M. The impact of past and present preferences on stimulus engagement in nursing home residents with dementia. Aging Ment Health. 2010;14(1):67–73.
22. Cohen-Mansfield J. The impact of environmental factors on persons with dementia attending recreational groups. Int J Geriatr Psychiatry. 2020;35(2):141–6.
23. Cohen-Mansfield J, Thein K, Dakheel-Ali M, Regier NG, Marx MS. The value of social attributes of stimuli for promoting engagement in persons with dementia. J Nerv Ment Dis. 2010;198(8):586–92.
24. Cohen-Mansfield J, Thein K, Marx MS, Dakheel-Ali M, Freedman L. Efficacy of nonpharmacologic interventions for agitation in advanced dementia: a randomized, placebo-controlled trial. J Clin Psychiatry. 2012;73(9):1255–61.
25. Ballard C, Corbett A, Orrell M, et al. Impact of person-centred care training and person-centred activities on quality of life, agitation, and antipsychotic use in people with dementia living in nursing homes: a cluster-randomised controlled trial. PLoS Med. 2018;15(2):e1002500.
26. McDermid J, Da Silva MV, Williams G, Khan Z, Corbett A, Ballard C. A randomized controlled trial of a digital adaptation of the WHELD person-centered nursing home training program. J Am Med Dir Assoc. 2022;23(7):1166–70.

The Spectrum of Delirium

10

Tiffany Long and Lindsay Wilson

Key Points

1. Delirium is common in older adults in the hospital and post-acute care and nursing home settings.
2. Delirium is highly underrecognized and leads to poor short- and long-term outcomes related to morbidity, mortality, and brain health.
3. The cause of delirium is multifactorial and involves a combination of predisposing and precipitating risk factors.
4. The best treatment of delirium is prevention, followed by identifying and treating the underlying causes.

10.1 Introduction

Delirium is a neuropsychiatric syndrome characterized by an acute, fluctuating, and reversible disturbance in brain function [1]. Delirium is common in older adults in a variety of healthcare settings and is associated with increased morbidity, mortality, functional decline, healthcare costs, and nursing home placement [2]. Despite these significant and sometimes long-term sequelae, delirium often goes unrecognized in clinical practice. Timely and accurate diagnosis is important to address reversible causes of delirium and reduce complications of delirium. Understanding the epidemiology and risk factors for delirium is paramount to prevention and treatment.

T. Long (✉) · L. Wilson
Division of Geriatrics, Department of Internal Medicine, University of North Carolina Chapel Hill, Chapel Hill, NC, USA
e-mail: Tiffany.long@unchealth.unc.edu; Lindsay.wilson@unchealth.unc.edu

E. L. Cobbs, C. P. Prather (eds.), *Diseases of the Mind*, Topics in Geriatric Care,
https://doi.org/10.1007/978-981-97-5995-8_10

10.2 Epidemiology

Delirium is one of the most frequent symptoms of disease in the elderly and is especially common in hospitalized older adults [3, 4]. Approximately one-third of patients 70 years or older who are hospitalized on general medical services have delirium. Among those undergoing elective surgery, the incidence is 15–25% [4]. Higher-risk surgeries, such as cardiac or hip fracture repair, carry an incidence closer to 50%. Older patients mechanically ventilated in the ICU have an incidence of 75%. Prevalence reaches 85% at the end of life [5].

Outside of the hospital, delirium occurs in up to 60% of patients in post-acute care settings and nursing homes. In communities, the overall prevalence of delirium is 1–2%, sharply rising to 14% in patients 85 years or older. The 1-year mortality rate associated with cases of delirium is 35–40% [6]. Hospital-associated complications are more likely to occur in patients with delirium and can worsen the course of delirium. Common hospital-associated complications include pressure injuries, deep vein thrombosis (DVT), pulmonary embolisms (PE), constipation, catheter-associated infections, deconditioning, functional decline, falls, malnutrition, and dehydration [4].

Despite delirium's profound clinical implications, it is often unrecognized by healthcare providers due to several factors: the course of symptoms in delirium fluctuates, the symptoms overlap with those symptoms of dementia, and the diagnosis requires a high index of suspicion and familiarity with bedside clinical diagnostic tools. Hyperactive delirium, the most easily recognized by providers, is characterized by agitation, while hypoactive delirium is marked by lethargy and decreased motor activity, which can mimic fatigue or sleepiness [6]. Hypoactive delirium accounts for up to 75% of delirium and is associated with a poor prognosis, likely because it often goes unrecognized [7, 8].

10.3 Diagnosis and Clinical Features

Delirium is an acute state of confusion marked by a disturbance in consciousness and attention that fluctuates with lucid intervals. Global cognition is impaired which may manifest as incoherent speech, hallucinations, or delusions [2]. There is a marked inability to concentrate and pay attention. These symptoms are a distinct change from the patient's baseline [9]. One of the most important steps in establishing the diagnosis is obtaining collateral history regarding the patient's baseline mental status from family and caregivers. The DSM V offers official diagnostic criteria as listed in Table 10.1. The Confusion Assessment Method (CAM) was developed by Inouye et al. [11] and is a highly sensitive, specific, and reliable assessment tool to diagnose delirium at the bedside. The diagnosis of delirium in this model is centered around four key features listed in Table 10.2 and illustrated in Fig. 10.1 [11].

Table 10.1 DSM V criteria for diagnosis of delirium [10]

Delirium diagnosis requires all the following criteria
Disturbance in attention and awareness
Disturbance develops acutely and fluctuates in severity
At least one additional disturbance in cognition
Disturbance is not better explained by preexisting dementia
Disturbance does not occur in the context of severely reduced level of arousal or coma
Evidence of underlying organic cause

Table 10.2 Confusion assessment method (CAM) [11]

Diagnosis of delirium requires both features 1 and 2 plus either feature 3 or 4
Feature 1: Acute onset and fluctuating course
Feature 2: Inattention
Feature 3: Disorganized thinking
Feature 4: Altered level of consciousness

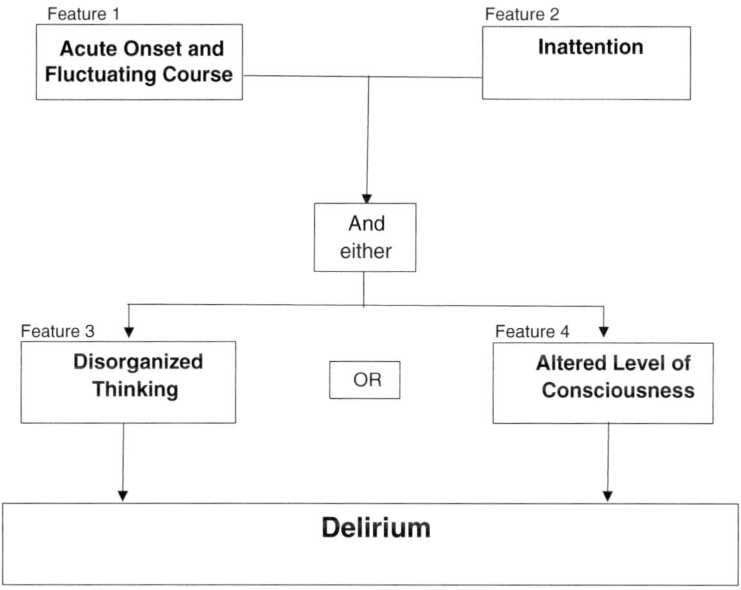

Fig. 10.1 Confusion assessment method

Once a diagnosis of delirium is determined, a thorough workup for underlying causes should be performed. This evaluation includes but is not limited to reviewing the medication list, evaluating for infection, urinary retention, constipation, and electrolyte disturbances, and performing a thorough physical examination.

10.4 Risk Factors for Delirium

Delirium is a multifactorial syndrome that is rarely caused by one single factor. The pathophysiology of delirium is not fully understood but is hypothesized to result from systemic inflammatory cytokine response and neurotransmitter disruption [12]. The development of delirium involves a complex interplay between baseline patient vulnerabilities, known as predisposing factors, and acute insults, known as precipitating factors [13]. When a patient has several predisposing factors, fewer precipitating factors are needed for delirium to occur. Conversely, when a patient has fewer predisposing factors, more precipitating factors are needed for delirium to develop. This model explains how a 90-year-old, frail patient with cognitive and sensory impairment may become delirious with an episode of constipation, while a 70-year-old patient with normal memory and excellent functional status would not (Table 10.3).

Table 10.3 Predisposing and precipitating factors [4, 14, 15]

Predisposing factors
Cognitive impairment
Older age
History of delirium
Depression
Hearing impairment
Visual impairment
Malnutrition
Immobility
Dependence on activities of daily living
Sleep deprivation
Precipitating factors
Drugs (sedative hypnotics, anticholinergic agents, anesthesia)
Surgery
Pain
Infection
Acute illness
Constipation
Urinary retention
Change in environment

10.5 Implications for Long-term Brain Health

A meta-analysis of delirium in the elderly showed that delirium is independently associated with a twofold risk of death, a 2.4-fold increased risk of institutionalization, and a 12.5-fold increased risk of dementia [16]. Delirium is also associated with a sustained decline in physical function, with an average loss of one activity of daily living per delirious episode [17]. A recent meta-analysis showed that delirium may be an independent risk factor for long-term cognitive decline in both surgical and nonsurgical patients. In every study, patients who experienced delirium displayed worse cognitive performance 3 months or longer after the episode [18]. Delirium serves both as a marker of decreased brain reserve and as a potential mechanism for permanent cognitive damage [15].

10.6 Management

Prevention of delirium is the most effective strategy to address delirium. In a landmark study in 1999, the Hospital Elder Life Program (HELP) intervened on six risk factors for delirium on inpatient general medicine units. These risk factors included cognitive impairment, sleep deprivation, immobility, visual impairment, hearing impairment, and dehydration. Interventions included providing reorientation, using a nonpharmacologic sleep protocol [19], getting the patient out of bed and walking, encouraging the use of eyeglasses and hearing aids, and promoting fluid intake. The incidence of delirium in the usual care group was 15% compared with 9.9% in the prevention group. The duration of delirium was also reduced in the prevention group as evidenced by the total 105 days of delirium compared to 161 days in the usual care group. These interventions significantly reduced the incidence and duration of episodes of delirium in patients 70 years or older [14].

Treatment of delirium involves identifying and addressing the underlying causes, such as discontinuing delirium-inducing medications, treating infection, correcting metabolic derangements, and addressing pain, urinary retention, and constipation. Close attention to environmental factors is important in delirium management. During the day, the room should be well-lit with natural light by keeping the window blinds open, and at night, the room should be dark and quiet. Sleep interruptions should be limited as much as possible. Patients should be encouraged and, if needed, helped out of bed and into a bedside chair frequently during the day. Family members should be directed to stay at the patient's bedside to reorient and reassure the patient. Eyeglasses and hearing aids should be used to reduce sensory deprivation. Finally, the medical team should adopt a proactive and aggressive approach to preventing hospital-associated complications.

10.7 High-Risk Medications in Delirium

Any medications that cause CNS depression or have anticholinergic properties increase the risk of delirium. A careful review of the patient's medication list is imperative when treating episodes of delirium, as offending medications should be discontinued or weaned. Older patients are at an increased risk of side effects and toxicities of these medications, given their reduced cognitive reserve and changes in liver and renal metabolism with age (Tables 10.4 and 10.5).

Table 10.4 Common anticholinergic side effects [20]

Decreased salivation
Decreased sweating
Dilated pupils
Urinary retention
Constipation
Blurred vision
Increased heart rate
Impaired concentration
Confusion
Attention deficit
Memory impairment

Table 10.5 High-risk medications in delirium [4, 19]

Drug class	Commonly prescribed medication names	Mechanism of adverse effect	Strategies for deprescribing
Benzodiazepines	Alprazolam	CNS sedation and withdrawal	If taking scheduled doses, they must be weaned slowly to prevent withdrawal; otherwise, they can discontinue
	Lorazepam		
	Diazepam		
	Clonazepam		
Sedative hypnotics	Zolpidem	CNS sedation and withdrawal	Can substitute with safer sleep aids including melatonin or lower the dose trazodone, implement non-pharmacologic sleep strategies including massage, warm drinks (milk, herbal tea), and relaxing music [19]
	Zaleplon		
Opioids	Oxycodone	Anticholinergic toxicity, CNS sedation	Introduce scheduled Tylenol, topical voltaren gel, lidocaine patches, joint injections, duloxetine. Reserve opioids for breakthrough pain. If on opioids, use lowest possible doses and work to slowly reduce the dose with the above measures
	Morphine		
	Hydromorphone		
	Fentanyl		

continued

Table 10.5 (Continued)

Drug class	Commonly prescribed medication names	Mechanism of adverse effect	Strategies for deprescribing
Anticholinergics	Oxybutynin Benztropine	Anticholinergic toxicity	Lower the dose and utilize scheduled toileting for urinary incontinence. Can also substitute less anticholinergic medications (mirabegron)
First-generation antihistamines	Diphenhydramine (Benadryl) Hydroxyzine	Anticholinergic toxicity	Discontinue and educate patients to avoid entirely. It should never be used as a sleep aid. Can substitute nasal sprays for nasal allergies or second-generation antihistamines for itching and full-body allergy symptoms (cetirizine, loratadine, and fexofenadine)
Tricyclic antidepressants	Nortriptyline Amitriptyline Imipramine Doxepin	Anticholinergic toxicity	Wean and replace with SSRIs for anxiety/depression. Consider duloxetine if indication is for chronic pain
Antipsychotics	Haloperidol Quetiapine Risperidone Olanzapine	CNS sedation, anticholinergic toxicity	Discontinue or use lower doses. Consider risk versus benefit in delirium

10.8 Pharmacological Management of Delirium

Pharmacologic management of delirium is reserved for cases of hyperactive delirium when the patient's behavior is dangerous to themselves or others or there are hallucinations or delusions that are causing the patient significant distress. A meta-analysis in 2016 reviewed 12 randomized control trials of antipsychotic agents for delirium and concluded there was no reduction in mortality, length of stay, and duration or severity of delirium [21]. The use of all medications for agitated delirium is off-label in the United States (Table 10.6).

Table 10.6 Pharmacotherapy options in hyperactive delirium [4, 21]

Medication	Medication class	Dosing (mg)	Routes	Degree of sedation	Risk of EPS	Comments
Haloperidol	Typical antipsychotic	0.25–1	Oral, IM, IV	Low	High	Monitor for QT prolongation, discuss risks versus benefits with health care agent
Risperidone	Atypical antipsychotic	0.25–0.5	Oral, IM	Low	High	Monitor for QT prolongation, discuss risks versus benefits with health care agent
Olanzapine	Atypical antipsychotic	2.5–5	Oral, sublingual, IM	Moderate	Moderate	Monitor for QT prolongation, discuss risks versus benefits with health care agent
Quetiapine	Atypical antipsychotic	12.5–25	Oral	High	Low	Preferred agent in patients with parkinsonism Monitor for QT prolongation, discuss risks versus benefits with health care agent
Lorazepam	Benzodiazepine	0.25–0.5	Oral, IM, IV	Very high	None	Only use in benzodiazepine withdrawal, catatonia, or alcohol withdrawal. Can worsen other forms of delirium
Trazodone	Antidepressant: SARI (serotonin antagonist and reuptake inhibitor)	12.5–25	Oral	Moderate	None	If used first line, can sometimes prevent use of antipsychotics

10.9 Conclusion

Delirium is common in older adults especially in the hospital, post-acute care, and nursing home settings. The risk of delirium rises with increasing age, increasing comorbidities, and cognitive impairment. Delirium can be life-threatening and is also associated with high morbidity and increased risk of long-term nursing home placement. Patients who have baseline brain vulnerability are both at an increased risk of developing delirium and having devastating long-term sequelae of delirium. Despite these serious consequences, delirium is often undiagnosed and mismanaged. Being able to quickly recognize delirium and rapidly identify and treat the underlying cause is imperative for physicians and healthcare workers in all healthcare settings. Prevention is possible, and strategies for prevention should be better implemented in high-risk settings. The pathophysiology of delirium is not fully understood given the heterogenous and multifactorial nature of the disease. There should be a larger emphasis on research for delirium as well as training healthcare workers on all levels of care to be able to prevent, identify, and manage delirium.

References

1. Grover S, Avasthi A. Clinical practice guidelines for management of delirium in elderly. Indian J Psychiatry. 2018;60(Suppl 3):S329–40. https://doi.org/10.4103/0019-5545.224473.
2. Arenson C, Busby-Whitehead J, Brummel-Smith K, Reichel W. Recognition and management of delirium. In: Reichel's care of the elderly clinical aspects of aging. 6th ed. Cambridge University Press; 2009. p. 171–5.
3. Bucht G, Gustafson Y, Sandberg O. Epidemiology of delirium. Dement Geriatr Cogn Disord. 1999;10(5):315–8. https://doi.org/10.1159/000017161.
4. Mercantonio ER. Delirium in hospitalized older adults. N Engl J Med. 2017;377:1456–66. https://doi.org/10.1056/NEJMcp1605501.
5. Marcantonio ER. Postoperative delirium: a 76-year-old woman with delirium following surgery. JAMA. 2012;308:73–81. https://doi.org/10.1001/jama.2012.6857.
6. Inouye SK. Delirium in older persons. N Engl J Med. 2006;354:1157–65. https://doi.org/10.1056/NEJMra052321.
7. Kiely DK, Jones RN, Bergmann MA, Marcantonio ER. Association between psychomotor activity delirium subtypes and mortality among newly admitted post-acute facility patients. J Gerontol A Biol Sci Med Sci. 2007;62:174–9. https://doi.org/10.1093/gerona/62.2.174.
8. Yang FM, Marcantonio ER, Inouye SK, et al. Phenomenological subtypes of delirium in older persons: patterns, prevalence, and prognosis. Psychosomatics. 2009;50:248–54. https://doi.org/10.1176/appi.psy.50.3.248.
9. Burns A, Gallagley A, Byrne J. Delirium. J Neurol Neurosurg Psychiatry. 2004;75(3):362–7. https://doi.org/10.1136/jnnp.2003.023366.
10. American Psychiatric Association DSM-5 Task Force. Diagnostic and statistical manual of mental disorders. 5th ed. Washington, DC: American Psychiatric Association; 2013.
11. Inouye SK, Inouye S, van Dyck C, Alessi C, Balkin S, Siegal A, Horwitz R. Clarifying confusion: the confusion assessment method. Ann Intern Med. 1990;113(12):941–8. https://doi.org/10.7326/0003-4819-113-12-941.
12. Van Gool WA, van de Beek D, Eikelenboom P. Systemic infection and delirium: When cytokines and acetylcholine collide. Lancet. 2010;375(9716):773–5. https://doi.org/10.1016/S0140-6736(09)61158-2.

13. Inouye SK, Charpentier PA. Precipitating factors for delirium in hospitalized elderly persons: predictive model and interrelationship with baseline vulnerability. JAMA. 1996;275:852–7. https://doi.org/10.1001/jama.1996.03530350034031.
14. Inouye SK, Bogardus ST Jr, Charpentier PA, et al. A multicomponent intervention to prevent delirium in hospitalized older patients. NEJM. 1999;340:669–76. https://doi.org/10.1056/NEJM199903043400901.
15. Inouye SK, Westendorp RGJ, Saczynski JS. Delirium in elderly people. Lancet. 2014;383(9920):911–22. https://doi.org/10.1016/S0140-6736(13)60688-1.
16. Witlox J, Eurelings LSM, de Jonghe JFM, et al. Delirium in elderly patients and the risk of postdischarge mortality, institutionalization, and dementia: a meta-analysis. JAMA. 2010;304:443–51. https://doi.org/10.1001/jama.2010.1013.
17. Murray AM, Levkoff SE, Wetle TT, et al. Acute delirium and functional decline in the hospitalized elderly patient. J Gerontol. 1993;48:M181–6.
18. Goldberg TE, Chen C, Wang Y, et al. Association of delirium with long-term cognitive decline: a meta-analysis. JAMA Neurol. 2020;77(11):1373–81. https://doi.org/10.1001/jamaneurol.2020.2273.
19. McDowell JA, Mion LC, Lydon TJ, Inouye SK. A nonpharmacologic sleep protocol for hospitalized older patients. J Am Geriatr Soc. 1998;46:700–5. https://doi.org/10.1111/j.1532-5415.1998.tb03803.x.
20. Lieberman JA. Managing anticholinergic side effects. Prim care companion. J Clin Psychiatry. 2004;6(Suppl 2):20–3.
21. Neufeld KJ, Yue J, Robinson TN, Inouye SK, Needham DM. Antipsychotic medication for prevention and treatment of delirium in hospitalized adults: a systematic review and meta-analysis. J Am Geriatr Soc. 2016;64:705–14. https://doi.org/10.1111/jgs.14076.

11 Supportive Decision-Making and Advance Care Planning

(Scott) Ian Borison and Sonika Pandey

Key Points

1. Advance care planning (ACP) should focus on the patient's preferences for decision-making, their values, beliefs, and prioritization of medical care.
2. ACP is a dynamic process that should be revisited and updated with changes in health or values.
3. A crucial component of ACP is determining appropriate surrogate decision-makers and including them in ACP discussions.
4. ACP discussions and advance directives should be incorporated into the electronic health record and made available to the entire healthcare team.

11.1 Background

Life expectancy in many parts of the world has grown significantly over the past few decades. The aging population will lead to increasing numbers of patients with chronic and life-limiting conditions. In the United States in 2020, four of the six leading causes of death were chronic and progressive illnesses: heart disease, cancer, chronic lower respiratory disease, and Alzheimer's disease [1]. In the United States, the prevalence of Alzheimer's dementia is about one in nine people over 65 years old [2].

(S.) I. Borison
Johns Hopkins University School of Medicine, Baltimore, MD, USA
e-mail: Sboriso2@jh.edu

S. Pandey (✉)
DC Veterans Affairs Hospital, George Washington University School of Medicine, Washington, DC, USA
e-mail: Sonika.Pandey@va.gov

E. L. Cobbs, C. P. Prather (eds.), *Diseases of the Mind*, Topics in Geriatric Care,
https://doi.org/10.1007/978-981-97-5995-8_11

Medical decision-making, especially in patients with life-limiting conditions, is inherently stressful for patients, their loved ones, and healthcare providers. Healthcare providers must be prepared to discuss difficult decisions with patients to provide care that reflects and aligns with their values, beliefs, and preferences.

A data review from the Health and Retirement Study showed that 70% of patients over 60 who required decision-making at the end of life lacked decision-making capacity. The presence of an advance directive can lead to care that is more aligned with a patient's preferences [3]. Advance directives can also benefit bereaved family members, who are less likely to report concerns with physician communication if an advance directive is present [4].

These facts and figures highlight the growing need for, and importance of, informed medical decision-making for geriatric patients.

11.2 Supportive Decision-Making

Supportive decision-making is extremely valuable in patients with dementia, where decision-making ability is expected to change over time. It is a collaborative process where the patient, their trusted surrogate, and healthcare provider discuss important aspects of their care and formulate a plan that most aligns with the patient's core values, goals and preferences [5].

Early discussions about current and future care preferences for patients with dementia allow for maximal participation from the patients. The involvement of a trusted surrogate should be encouraged throughout the trajectory. Discussions should focus on a values assessment to understand what matters most to the patient, what gives their life meaning, and what worries or concerns they have in the context of their illness. This will help to build rapport while giving perspective on how to best guide the patient's care now and in the future. Patients with dementia at the margins of decision-making capacity should be assisted by a surrogate when making decisions, and providers should make all efforts to deliver information in clear and simple terms.

11.3 Capacity Evaluation

A capacity evaluation may be required prior to addressing decision-making if there are concerns that a patient may not be able to make their own decisions. It is important to contrast capacity with competency. Competency is a global determination of decision-making ability and is a legal declaration. Capacity refers to the patient's ability to make a specific decision at a specific point in time. Medical providers can determine capacity, but they cannot determine competency.

Determining capacity may be a daunting task in practice; however, the general principles are not complex. A patient must be able to convey an understanding of the decision at hand and the potential consequences of their choices. The patient must be able to express their choice and provide logical reasoning for that choice.

Capacity does not require the practitioner to agree with the decision in principle, but it does require the patient to provide reasoning for their decision.

Decision-making capacity should always be assumed to be intact unless there is evidence to the contrary. Capacity should be determined on a decision-by-decision basis. Even if the patient exhibits poor cognitive function, they may have the capacity for less complicated decisions, such as naming a surrogate, but could lack the capacity for more complex decisions, such as discontinuing disease-directed therapy. If there is doubt that the patient has decision-making capacity, a formal assessment should be completed.

11.4 Facilitating a Discussion to Formulate an Individualized Plan

Developing an individualized care plan for patients with serious or progressive illness requires an understanding of the patient's values and goals in relation to their clinical situation. This process frequently includes discussing difficult news, eliciting patient's values, and providing thoughtful recommendations.

11.5 Discussing Difficult News: Adapted from the SPIKES Mnemonic as Published by Baile et al. [6]

11.5.1 Set Up and Setting

11.5.1.1 Set Up for the Meeting

Prior to meeting with a patient and their loved ones, consider discussing the clinical situation with any relevant consultants and determine potential options for a treatment plan. Consider the various treatment options and what information about the patient may be helpful to formulate the best recommendation. For instance, would a better understanding of how the patient prioritizes independence compared to longevity of life be helpful for the discussion?

11.5.1.2 Setting

Ensure a quiet and private location for the discussion with the appropriate stakeholders present. Determine the patient's preferences for decision-making. Do they prefer to make decisions on their own or with the help of others?

11.5.2 Perception: Assess the Patient's Understanding

Before providing information, it is important to gauge the patient's understanding of the current clinical situation. This may significantly impact the direction of the conversation as the patient may have a very advanced or limited understanding of their condition. Having a sense of the patient's perception can help the provider determine where to begin.

11.5.3 Invitation and Information Preferences

11.5.3.1 Information Preferences

Prior to providing new information to the patient, explore how they like information delivered. Do they prefer to know all the details or are they content with a big picture approach?

11.5.3.2 Invitation: Ask permission

Asking for an invitation to share knowledge is not only considerate, but it can also prepare the patient for the coming information and discussion.

11.5.4 Knowledge: Provide Knowledge

Consider a "warning shot" such as "The imaging did not show what we were hoping for." Then, provide information in concise, simple, and meaning-based terms. For example, "Unfortunately, the scan shows that your cancer has spread to many parts of your body, and this means that your cancer cannot be cured."

11.5.5 Emotion/Empathy: Expect and Address Emotion

After providing difficult news, patients will need time to process it. In these uncomfortable situations, one reflex is to explain the information further. Allow for a silent moment so that the patient may respond in whatever manner they choose. Providers should expect an emotional response after delivering difficult news. This is an opportunity to respond with empathy.

11.5.6 Strategy: Devise a Strategy for Next Steps

Spend time eliciting the patient's values in the context of the new information. Use this information to align your recommendation for the next steps with the hopes, values, and wishes of the patient.

11.6 Values Assessment

After providing relevant information to patients, elicit their personal values to help guide your recommendations. This should be accomplished with the use of open-ended questions. Common topics to discuss include values that have guided previous medical decisions, religious/spiritual beliefs, acceptable quality of life, etc.

It can be helpful to gauge a patient's prioritization of potentially competing values, such as how they balance quality of life versus prolongation of life. A difficult but sometimes revealing question is, "Can you imagine a quality of life that may be worse than death?" Other value-based questions to consider can be found in Box 11.1.

Box 11.1 Abstract Questions That Can Help to Elicit Values and Preferences

If you were faced with a decision of having more time (weeks or short months) with most of your time in a healthcare setting versus *less time (days or weeks) at home, which would you prefer?*

If time became short, what would be most important to you for your care?

What are your biggest worries?

What are you hoping for?

Do you have any spiritual beliefs or customs that would be important for your doctors to consider while caring for you?

11.7 Recommendations

Patients facing difficult decisions usually about their healthcare prefer to make decisions with guidance from their healthcare team. Providing a menu style of options without a recommendation can place patients in an uncertain position without clear direction. Providers may sometimes avoid making recommendations due to fear of overly paternalistic care. Asking for an invitation to provide a recommendation reinforces that the patient is still the ultimate decision-maker while also providing expert guidance. Informing the patient that regardless of their decisions, the care team will continue to support them and care for them builds the therapeutic alliance as well.

For further information on this process, visit the Serious Illness Care Program (https://www.ariadnelabs.org/serious-illness-care).

11.8 Advance Care Planning

Communication regarding serious illness does not only need to occur when there are pressing decisions to be made. Advance care planning (ACP) allows a patient to make decisions and guide their care in anticipation of decision-making needs. This can be exceptionally helpful for patients and their loved ones when facing a diagnosis of dementia, where their decision-making ability is expected to be affected over time.

Determining the patient's understanding of their disease, prognosis, and predicted disease trajectory and sharing information in this respect should precede discussions about future care. However, ACP should be discussed early in the disease to allow for maximal participation by the patient.

ACP is a dynamic and ongoing process that should be revisited periodically, as preferences and values can change with time [7, 8]. Even in the setting of dynamic capacity in dementia, patients should be included in discussions about values and care as this will provide helpful information and guidance for surrogates. There are many triggers that prompt initial ACP discussions and revisiting ACP discussions (Fig. 11.1).

1. General
    a. Annual Wellness Exam
    b. Change in functional status or level of care
    c. Following hospitalization, or sub-acute rehabilitation discharge
    d. Patient requesting prognostic information or information regarding advance care planning
    e. Change in family or social situation, such as death of previously designated healthcare surrogate
2. Dementia
    a. On routine visit following diagnosis
    b. Changes in health status
    c. Upon establishment of Power of Attorney for finance/personal welfare
    d. Recurrent infections
    e. Functional decline
    f. Recurrent falls
3. Surprise question: Would you be surprised if the patient died within the next 6 months?

Fig. 11.1 Triggers for discussing ACP

The most important aspects of ACP are electing surrogate decision-makers and exploring values and preferences with patients to help guide future care [9]. This may include preferences regarding life-sustaining treatment interventions such as cardiopulmonary resuscitation, invasive ventilatory support, artificial nutrition, or other disease-specific interventions. Electronic medical records should have a designated section to document ACP discussions and advance directives to allow easy access.

ACP that focuses on the goals, values, and beliefs of patients has been shown in randomized trials to improve the likelihood that their end-of-life wishes are known and followed [10]. Trials have also shown positive impacts on family members, including less stress, anxiety, and depression [10, 11].

11.9 Advance Directives

An advance directive is a legal document with a written statement of a patient's wishes regarding medical care to ensure their wishes are followed even if they lack capacity. Prepare for Your Care (www.prepareforyourcare.org) and Five Wishes (www.fivewishes.org) are resources for completing advance directives.

11.10 Living Will

A living will is a type of advance directive which specifies which medical treatments the patient finds acceptable or unacceptable. It can also address preferences for organ donation or human body donation.

11.11 Durable Power of Attorney

Advance directives usually outline a durable power of attorney (DPOA), which designates a person to make decisions on the patient's behalf if the patient is incapacitated. Patients can elect either an individual or a group of people as a surrogate for healthcare decisions. This is separate from electing a financial surrogate.

If no surrogate is chosen, the patient is potentially leaving medical decisions to their next of kin or a court-appointed surrogate, depending on local laws. Electing a DPOA can be especially meaningful for marginalized patients and those with non-traditional families, such as members of the LGBTQ+ community.

11.12 How to Translate ACP into Advance Directives

Advance care planning discussions may lead to the completion of an advance directive. Patients may bring advance directives to their healthcare provider to review or ask for assistance; however, providers should be prepared to initiate this process. When guiding patients with ACP and completing advance directives, it is not necessary to decide yes or no for each potential intervention. The most important aspect of these documents is to determine the values that guide the patient's decision-making. Potential surrogates should be invited to these discussions, as these discussions can help guide decisions if the patient becomes incapacitated.

In the setting of provider or patient uncertainty over decisions regarding specific treatments, such as invasive mechanical ventilation, it is reasonable to recommend a time-limited trial. An AHRQ study found that patients were more likely to accept short-term mechanical ventilation than long-term ventilation regardless of health state [12]. If a time-limited trial is selected, then it can be helpful to determine a reasonable time frame for the intervention.

11.13 Conclusion

Supportive decision-making and ACP help ensure patients' healthcare matches their values and wishes. Supportive decision-making includes engaging loved ones to assist patients with dynamic capacity in healthcare decisions. This process also includes evaluating a patient's perception of their health, sharing information about their health, completing a values assessment, and providing thoughtful recommendations. ACP is a dynamic process that should be adapted to changes in a patient's health and changes in a patient's priorities and values. The first step in ACP is determining a suitable surrogate or DPOA. ACP should prioritize gaining an understanding of how a patient makes healthcare decisions and what values guide these decisions. When possible, the patient's loved ones and potential surrogates should be invited to these discussions. Documentation of these discussions should be placed in the electronic health record with an emphasis on the patient's values.

References

1. CDC Fast Stats. 19 Sept 2022. https://www.cdc.gov/nchs/fastats/leading-causes-of-death.htm.
2. 2022 Alzheimer's Disease Facts and Figures. Special report: more than normal aging: understanding mild cognitive impairment. Alzheimer's Association. https://www.alz.org/media/Documents/alzheimers-facts-and-figures.pdf.
3. Silveria MJ, Kim SYH, Langa KM. Advance directives and outcomes of surrogate decision making before death. N Engl J Med. 2010;362:1211–8.
4. Teno JM, Gruneir A, Schwartz Z, et al. Association between advance directives and quality of end-of- life care: a national study. J Am Geriatr Soc. 2007;55:189–94.
5. Dening KH, Sampson EL, De Vries K. Advance care planning in dementia: recommendations for healthcare professionals. Palliat Care. 2019;12:1178224219826579.
6. Baile WF, Buckman R, Lenzi R, et al. SPIKES—a six-step protocol for delivering bad news: application to the patient with cancer. Oncologist. 2000;5(4):302–11. https://doi.org/10.1634/theoncologist.5-4-302.
7. Lum HD, Sudore RL, Bekelman DB. Advance care planning in the elderly. Med Clin North Am. 2015;99(2):391–403.
8. Piers R, Albers G, Gilissen J, et al. Advance care planning in dementia: recommendations for healthcare professionals. BMC Palliat Care. 2018;17:88.
9. Bernacki R, Block S. Communication about serious illness care goals: a review and synthesis of best practices. JAMA Intern Med. 2014;174(12):1994–2003.
10. Detering KM, Hancock AD, Reade MC, Silvester W. The impact of advance care planning on end of life care in elderly patients: randomized controlled trial. BMJ. 2010;340:c1345.
11. Wright AA, Zhang B, Ray A, et al. Associations between end-of-life discussions, patient mental health, medical care near death and caregiver bereavement adjustment. JAMA. 2008;300(14):1665–73.
12. Advance care planning: preferences for care at the end of life. Research in Action—AHRQ. Department of Health & Human Services. Issue 12, 2003.

Correction to: Dementia Syndromes

Elizabeth Clark, Rachael Kantor, and Sophie Lin

Correction to:
Chapter 8 in: E. L. Cobbs, C. P. Prather (eds.), *Diseases of the Mind*, Topics in Geriatric Care, https://doi.org/10.1007/978-981-97-5995-8_8

The first name of Rachael Kantor was unfortunately published with an error. The initially published version has now been corrected.

The updated version of this chapter can be found at
https://doi.org/10.1007/978-981-97-5995-8_8

E. L. Cobbs, C. P. Prather (eds.), *Diseases of the Mind*, Topics in Geriatric Care,
https://doi.org/10.1007/978-981-97-5995-8_12

MIX
Papier aus verantwortungsvollen Quellen
Paper from responsible sources
FSC® C105338

If you have any concerns about our products, you can contact us on
ProductSafety@springernature.com

In case Publisher is established outside the EU, the EU authorized representative is:
Springer Nature Customer Service Center GmbH
Europaplatz 3, 69115 Heidelberg, Germany

Printed by Libri Plureos GmbH
in Hamburg, Germany